Facing Up

A Patient's Guide
to Healing the Face

by

Lois Hawk Todd

Published by:
Capuchin Post
PO Box 1388
Paonia, CO 81428

First Edition © 2016 by Lois Hawk Todd
ISBN 978-1517701994

Printed in the United States of America
Interior designed by Mary C Simmons, set in Garamond
Cover design and background photo by Mary C Simmons

ACKNOWLEDGEMENTS

Throughout the long journey of my healing, my husband, Allen Todd and son, Ryan Todd, were a source of love and support. Thanks, guys.

So many friends and family stepped forward to help, they are too numerous to mention, yet I would be remiss in not acknowledging Janice Madariaga, who rallied the troops after my accident and organized kind and most welcomed care from my community. A thank you, also, to my god-parents, Janet and Deacon David Fabula, for their help. My friend Margaret Crawford has taught me more about life than anyone I know. For that, and all the fun - thank you, Mz. Margaret.

My journey was blessed with good doctors and medical folk. Top of the list is my guru doctor, Dr. Frederick Menick of Tucson, Arizona. His amazing talent, along with his concentrated care, make him a miracle worker in my book. My sincere thanks to Dr. George MooYoung, my retinologist, whose compassion and humility continue to inspire me. Finally, thank you to my Trekkie family; those crazy folks who filled difficult days with love and laughter. My PJ Pals — Francine Lebrato and Lisa Bailey, David and Alicia Ivy, "My Captain" David Williams, "My Date" Guy Davidson, and all the other wonderful folks of my Trek World; I appreciate you more than you can know.

May we live long and prosper.

Cover photographs
Begin at upper left, counter clockwise to center photo

1. February 1995. This is my original face. The photo was taken a year and a half before my accident where I was struck in the face by an eighty-five mile an hour baseball while wearing glasses.

2. July 1998. This photo was taken two years after my accident and fifteen months after completion of subsequent surgeries. The damage to my pupil left it fully dilated and oddly shaped. Also noticeable is the depression of my left cheek.

3. August 2006. This was taken two weeks before my cancer removal. Working to synchronize the muscles in my face, wearing glasses and weight gain all helped increase the symmetry of my face.

4. August 2006. The extensive scar tissue from my accident turned to basal cell carcinoma. Via Mohs, a surgical cancer removal system, more than twenty per cent of my face was removed to rid it of the cancer. This photo was shot post-flap down and skin rearrangement surgery, which covered the hole the Mohs created.

5. July 2008. After completing five surgeries as a result of my cancer, my doctor and insurance company determined this was an adequate appearance. I did not agree. I felt deformed. I sought the expertise of a rhino-plastic surgeon in Tucson, AZ.

6. June 2009. This was taken after completing the first surgery with my Tucson doctor in which he built my nose. The alar was not formed until his second surgery

7. January 2012. This was taken just before my final surgery in Tucson. My left eye had been eviscerated in 2010. I now wear a prosthetic eye.

8. August 2015. My new face; this photo was taken after completion of my third facial reconstruction. (Photo credit: Ann Marie Gambino)

TABLE OF CONTENTS

INTRODUCTION

How I Got into This Predicament

July 28, 1996: Baseball—like many Little League families, it consumed our lives. On this particular day, my husband Allen, my ten-year-old son Ryan and I were at the batting cages. Officially, we were there for Ryan to practice but as was often the case, a competition flared up between my husband and me.

At the time, I was quite athletic. I played racquetball weekly and though I had no baseball experience, my batting swing was brutally accurate. Allen and I progressed up the ball speeds to the eighty-five mile-per-hour pitch. Watching him go up against that kind of speed was both frightening and exhilarating. He managed to hit a few.

I stepped into the cage, knowing I would do the same. My excitement turned to frustration. The machine wasn't working. We called for help and soon a man began repairing the batting machine. I stepped out of the batter's box but stayed in the cage. Allen and Ryan were on the other side of the fence and we bantered about my pending performance.

Then, something made me turn. In a split second, I saw a ball roaring toward me. It was the last thing I saw with any accuracy out of my left eye. The impact whirled me around like a top. I went down to my knees. Blood poured from my face like an open faucet.

People shouted. Hands grabbed me; my husband's, others'. It was a mad fight to stop the bleeding. I heard my son screaming. I wanted to comfort him. I tried yelling, but everything was too loud, too chaotic. "I found her glasses," someone said. I knew my eye was gone, but I fought not to think about it.

Blood kept pouring and I feared I would bleed to death. Finally, the ambulance arrived. As they wheeled me out of the park, I remember looking up at a giant cottonwood tree shimmering in the breeze and thinking, "How could this happen on such a beautiful day?"

The damage was extensive. My eye was saved and for that, I will always be thankful, but it was not the same eye I awoke with that morning. Forty-two stitches closed a hole in the front of the eye and in the back, the retina was detached. Once my eye was stabilized, people asked me "What kind of vision do you have with that eye?" Like all things, it was a matter of perspective.

A "seeing" person would find it a disorienting nuisance because what little vision I had created double vision, but having had a father who ended his life blind (a victim of glaucoma), I knew that any and all sight was valuable. In the beginning, my left eye vision was enough that I could see my way out of a room. It would have been slow progress. I would have bumped into things, but I could have made it. To some people, it would be a wonderful gift.

My eye was just the beginning of the damage. The impact of the ball had shattered my face. My nose was pushed to the right, the bone below the eye depressed, cheekbone broken, orbital bone broken and a tripod break, which basically shifted all the bones below my eye. Nine months and five surgeries later, I was put back together—not the same as I was before, of course.

The eye, that ever so noticeable lamp of the soul, especially for a blue-eyed person like me, was what you noticed first. My pupil remained fully dilated and had an odd, almost catlike, shape. Next to be noticed was the asymmetry of my bone structure. The area to the side of my nose and below the eye was depressed. The left cheekbone was a bit lower and more protruding than the right. My left eyebrow was lower than the right and the lid tended to droop. There was nerve damage. My left upper lip drooped and there were those embarrassing moments when I was unaware that my nose was running because I have little feeling in my left nostril. The scarring was extensive. Most of the left side of my nose and much of the area beside and under my eye were heavily scarred—a pale, burn victim look.

However, as time went on, I learned to accept my new look. I developed techniques to maximize my appearance and, once again, I felt like a reasonably attractive woman.

The people around me were a tremendous help in my healing process. I lived in a very small town and everyone in our valley seemed involved in making Lois well again.

As I stated, my accident was in July but it was not until September that I knew my left eye could be saved. During that time, my eye seemed on everyone's mind and I truly believe their prayers and well wishes made a big difference in my healing. I heard encouraging words almost daily.

"You look fine." "You're doing great." The first twenty days after my accident I did not have to cook a single meal. Each night someone would show up on my doorstep with a prepared dish. How can you not heal under such compassionate circumstances?

I had five surgeries over a nine-month period due to my accident:

JULY 28, 1996

The front of my eye was repaired, requiring forty-two stitches. My nose was put back in position. I received a blood transfusion due to excessive blood loss.

AUGUST 4, 1996

Repair of an arterial cut in my nose. An ear, nose and throat doctor packed my nose, hoping the arterial cut would heal itself. When the nurse pulled the packing seven days after my accident, the artery had not repaired. I lost over a pint of blood before she managed to stop the bleeding. I am still angry that the cut was not repaired that first day. I refused to see that doctor again and continue to recommend others avoid him.

SEPTEMBER 10, 1996

My retina was reattached and my lens removed.

JANUARY 15, 1997

My sinuses were repaired and my nose aligned better.

APRIL 4, 1997

I had an orbital blowout repair in which a plate was put under my eye to replace the broken bone. My doctors wanted to do further cosmetic work, but I had had enough. I wanted life, not more surgery.

As time went on, the accident became a memory. The things in my life that had changed—my appearance, the loss of vision in my left eye, the consequences of head injury—became a part of me. Yet, at times, I would remember something about the accident or surgeries and I would get a terrible feeling. How did I survive it, I wondered. I knew I could never go through something like that again.

Yet, I did.

On the tenth anniversary of my accident, I learned all my scar tissue had turned to basal cell carcinoma.

My face was ripped into again.

I reached out for support after my accident, but I withdrew with my basal cell carcinoma (BCC). Part of it was changes in me. At the time of my accident, I was outgoing, always looking for the company of others. By the time of the BCC diagnosis, I was a different person. I was still described as outgoing and talkative, but in truth, I had become a private person, generally preferring time alone. Yet, there was more than my desire for privacy in keeping the BCC to myself.

I didn't want anyone to know I had BCC. I wanted it to slip by unnoticed. The few people I told prior to my surgical odyssey were mostly clerks and tellers that I saw frequently and didn't want to startle with my pending appearance. "I won't be looking too good next time you see me," I warned. Most of my friends and family I didn't even tell. I wrote my Uncle Con's children only out of concern for them. We had lost Uncle Con the year before and my plan was to be there for my cousins during that painful first anniversary of his death. I wrote and told them that I would be recouping from surgery but I would be with them in spirit. They wrote back very worried about "my cancer." I never called it cancer. It was basal cell carcinoma, a completely different thing in my book. Cancer was that Oh-My-God-I-might-die-shoot-me-full-of-poison-puke-my-guts-out thing. I had a growth, an annoying lump that would soon be removed with no need for further treatment. Just one quick slice and it would be gone—forever and ever and ever.

I admit it. Not only did cancer scare the hell out of me, I was ashamed to have it. A condemning finger was pointed. "What did you do wrong?" It's my cells in my body. Every bit of the problem is inside me, so I must have really screwed up. Or maybe I had bad genes. Bad genes: it's like being the dumb kid in class, mean old Mrs. Samuelson glaring down at you, "What's wrong with you? Why have you failed so miserably?" Ugly, shameful, wicked stuff, cancer.

There is nothing heroic about it. The accident was different. Out of nowhere, I was attacked. My husband encircled me with trembling arms. Complete strangers worked to save me in the authoritative chaos of rescue by ambulance. It was the kind of thing you see in the news; "local hero" "valiant effort."

There is nothing heroic about cancer—except getting through it.

My diagnosis was slow in coming. I had been receiving Marie Katelle facials. The scar tissue on my face, which had been clear, lifeless, and rupturing easily, began to perk up and look healthy. Then bumps like pimples began to appear. A few that came to heads seemed to have little fragments come out of them, but one lump would not come to a head.

I went to a dermatologist, and he thought the best treatment would be to inject steroids to reduce its size. I would not agree to the treatment. Not only did I hate the thought of steroids, I knew I wanted the lump removed, so he sent me to another doctor. He was a plastic surgeon. He gave the same advice, but when I insisted the lump should be removed, he ordered an X-ray to see if anything was inside the lump.

The X-ray showed possible foreign material but was not conclusive. The plastic surgeon then suggested I see one of the doctors who treated me after my accident. I went to see the ear, nose and throat doctor who had performed two of my surgeries: the nose/artery repair and the nose/sinus repair. I had been impressed with his work. He now also specialized in plastic surgery. He scarcely looked at my face before saying he thought I had BCC and took samples for a biopsy. He said that judging from the area involved I would need to have a surgery in which a flap of skin from my forehead would be brought down to cover my nose. He said the surgery might make me look better.

After the biopsy came back positive, I was scheduled for two immediate surgeries; first with a dermatologist to remove the cancer and then with the ear, nose and throat doctor, now also a plastic surgeon, to begin reconstruction. I did not meet the dermatologist until the day of surgery, though I spoke with him on the phone. I did not see my plastic surgeon again until after the Mohs surgery.

My BCC surgeries and reconstruction with the ear, nose and throat doctor included five surgeries over a sixteen-month period:

August 30, 2006

Mohs removal of cancer. Mohs is a machine that tests the cancer as you go so when you walk out of the office, you know it's gone. My appointment began at 9:30 a.m. It didn't ended until 9:00 p.m., in part because the doctor was overbooked, but also because the cancer was far more extensive than expected. Pre-op estimates had been a 2.8 x 3.0 cm area, but what was removed was 4.5 x 5.0 cm. In total, more than twenty percent of my face was taken. The area removed began at the top of my nose, going down the bridge then out into the left cheek approximately one and one quarter inches then up to the top of the nose again and including most of the area under my eye. Much of the tissue was removed to the bone.

September 5, 2006

Flap down and skin rearrangement. It was as diabolical as it sounds. Having a gaping hole in my face, I needed it covered. A flap of skin from my scalp, still attached by a length of skin from my forehead (like an umbilical cord), was placed on my nose. To cover the remaining hole, I was cut from the upper ear, across to the orbital bone then under the eye to the nose and down the cheek to the chin. My skin was then pulled to cover the remaining hole. This meant that after losing twenty percent of my face, an additional fifty percent of what remained was severely shifted—brutal but effective.

OCTOBER 17, 2006

Flap removal. The skin serving as the umbilical cord was removed. (I called it my Ferengi butthead—if you are a Star Trek fan, you'll get this.)

MAY 14, 2007

My left eye ended up quite a bit lower than the right eye, so my eyelid next to my nose was raised and further work done on the "butthead" area.

DECEMBER 11, 2007

This time the other side of my eyelid was lifted allowing my left eye to appear more level. In addition, I had a "lift" to alleviate some of the excess skin on my left cheek. This completed my surgeries by this doctor.

I was not pleased with my looks. My face was very asymmetrical, I was heavily scarred, I had excess skin at my cheek, my eye protruded. To me, I looked deformed.

I decided I was unwilling to live with my appearance and, thus, decided to seek a third facial reconstruction. Fortunately, I found a doctor in Tucson, Arizona who is one of the finest rhinoplasty surgeons in the United States. I quickly dubbed him my guru doctor.

Over a three-year period, I went through five surgeries while under his care. In the midst of these surgeries, my left eye was eviscerated. This was caused by my accident, not the cancer.

When my retina was reattached fourteen years prior, the retinologist predicted my eye would last ten years. It lasted fourteen years. Though losing my eye was sad, it had become nearly sightless and very painful. The surgery was done by a Denver occuloplastic surgeon. Eviscerating my eye in October of 2010 was a relief.

January 2, 2009.

My first surgery with my guru doctor in Tucson. Essentially, all surgical areas were reopened and corrected. A large scar area on my scalp from which the flap skin had been taken, was repaired. My forehead was reopened and realigned, to appear less crooked.

The "butthead" area was corrected and he moved my right eyebrow into a more natural position—my right eyebrow had been pulled to the center of my brow by previous surgery. In addition, he removed a large scar on the side of my nose that protruded outward, as well as into the septum.

He reset the flap, so it looked natural and healthy, thus, ending the "Band-Aid" appearance. To correct my snarling look, he built a nostril with ear cartilage and lowered the left side of the nose to match the right.

He also began building an alar—the alar is the edge

of the nostril that flares. At the time of this surgery, I didn't have an alar on my left side.

He removed excess skin from my cheek and put in a smile line on my left side to match the right side. The second surgery with my guru doctor was on June 10, 2009. He completed the alar and extended my nose. He did further touch up on my cheek.

June 12, 2009

My third surgery. My lower left lid was very tight and aside from looking bad, the tightness made my eyelashes grow into my eye, causing irritation and damage to the cornea. My guru doctor arranged for me to have surgery with an occuloplastic surgeon in Tucson. She did a skin graft to my left lower lid using skin from my ear. This elevated the tightness.

May 17, 2011

I had another surgery with the Denver occuloplastic doctor who eviscerated my eye. He repaired the drooping of my left lid, giving my eye better alignment. Also, it helped me close my eyelid. After being fitted with my prosthetic eye, my lid wasn't able to fully close until this surgery.

He did further work on the "butthead" and my forehead scar. He then lifted my right eyelid to match the left better.

January 5, 2012

My final surgery. I think of this as my "putting on the chrome" surgery. My guru doctor in Tucson did a bit of touch up to my left cheek, my nose and the area to the left of my left eye. He also performed a face-lift to get the left and right sides of my face to match better. I looked a bit younger, too.

After sixteen surgeries to my face, I am thankful, relieved and over-joyed to say—I am done.

My next journey was writing a book on healing. My resume includes no medical background, but instead, hours logged in the trenches—a lot of hours. I hope my experience can help others learn to heal.

Oddly, healing is the one subject I felt lacking from my doctors and other medical professionals. They told me what drugs to take, how to change a bandage, they even provided lists of do's and don'ts, but they did not tell me how to heal.

A surgeon's scalpel cuts not just into a face but also into a person. The journey back can be, and to me should be, not just the body repaired but rather the healing of self—body, mind and soul.

It is with this belief I offer the following.

BEGINNING YOUR JOURNEY

CHAPTER 1

Choosing Your Doctor

The diagnosis is in. For whatever reason, your face is about to be invaded. What is your first step in the journey ahead? Choosing your doctor.

Your choice is important. When it comes to facial reconstruction, the difference from one doctor's work to another can be dramatic. I suppose this is true of all surgeons, but with facial surgery, every snip and decision is on public display. As a patient, you want to make sure the one holding the knife does a good job.

For my accident—an emergency situation—my doctor was the luck of the draw and I got lucky. My initial surgeon, an ophthalmologist who put my eye back together, was excellent and as work was needed outside his expertise, he referred me to equally good doctors. Ten years later, when my cancer was diagnosed, I went to a doctor I trusted and who had done a good job on my nose and sinuses after my accident. He was an ear, nose and throat doctor who now specialized in plastic surgery. As I stated in the introduction, he was the doctor who diagnosed my cancer when two other doctors failed. The only other doctor I contacted about surgery was a highly recommended dermatologist out of the University of Colorado. I decided against seeing him because his first available appointment was too far off. Besides, I trusted the ear, nose and throat doctor, and since he was now specializing in plastic surgery, he seemed a good choice. When he told me once my cancer was removed and reconstruction completed, I might look better, I felt confident.

I did not end up looking better. After completing a series of five surgeries with him, I felt deformed. In my doctor's defense, no one guessed my cancer was so extensive. The pre-op diagnosis size was 2.8 x 3.0 cm while the post-op size was 4.5 x 5.0 cm. When my doctor completed the flap down, his initial reconstruction surgery, he told my husband I was his biggest challenge to date—not very comforting news.

You may wonder why I didn't walk down the street and enlist the expertise of another doctor. We live in the boondocks. I didn't believe there was another doctor, unless I traveled outside our area, something I was not willing to do at that time. Besides, the ear, nose and throat doctor was confident about being up to the challenge and he had done well by me in previous surgeries.

What should I, the patient, have done differently? Research. One of my pet peeves is gossip. I hate it. Yet, in the search for a good reconstructive surgeon, I think gossip is just what you need. What do patients say about this doctor? Any complaints? (Inevitable.) Any gushing recommendations? What do other professionals have to say? The doctor should have photographs available, too, tangible evidence of his skills. Also, he should be board certified, which assures you he has had extensive training.

After my initial cancer surgeries, I learned the ear, nose and throat doctor and his office had changed in the ten years since my accident. The changes I saw were not good; yet, they were common. Patients were rushed through, the clock always ticking. Physician's assistants, whom I believed sometimes knew less than they thought they did, were taking the role of doctor. Insurance companies weighed in heavier than the patients themselves. The patient, bumped around this odd hierarchy, could slip through the cracks because the buck of patient responsibility never seemed to stop. The lack of information I received from the ear, nose and throat doctor caused problems for me. I became so frustrated that I contacted the dermatologist from the University of Colorado at his office in the town of Basalt.

I need to give a shout out here. When I called to make an appointment, I was frustrated beyond belief. Gertrude from his office spent twenty minutes explaining the ins and outs of my situation and calming me. I remember crying for half an hour after I hung up; I was so relieved to finally have straight and thorough answers.

While the Basalt doctor became my dermatologist, it was decided I would continue reconstruction with the ear, nose and throat doctor. A fifth surgery with him found me more or less a finished product.

I was far from happy with my looks. On many occasions, people asked me about the bandage on my nose. It was the skin flap. My left nostril was higher than the right, making me look like I was snarling.

There was a lot of scar tissue on my nose and it partially blocked my septum. My right eyebrow was pulled so far to the left, it now began at the center of my brow. I had excess skin on my cheek/jowl that sagged. The scar on my forehead was very noticeable and my face was crooked.

I looked deformed; I felt deformed. I asked my dermatologist who could help me. He suggested two plastic surgeons in all of the United States. I chose the one in Tucson, Arizona. Best decision I ever made. It took five additional surgeries, three with my Tucson plastic surgeon and two with occuloplastic surgeons, but I no longer feel deformed.

When searching for a doctor, do your homework. Shop around. Though most Americans are limited by their health insurance, most insurance companies have several doctors to choose from and at worst, you can consider paying more out of pocket expense to get the doctor you want. Even if your preferred doctor is cost prohibitive, get a consultation with him. He may give you ideas and insight to share with your surgeon. A tip: I found the cheaper the consultation fee, the better the doctor.

Get the opinion of another physician if you become disillusioned with your doctor and change doctors if you feel it necessary. As I said, I began seeing my dermatologist after being frustrated with the ear, nose and throat doctor. In doing so, I gained a lot of information. I felt more confident because a second pair of eyes were watching me. I think knowing another physician was watching made the ear, nose and throat doctor a bit more attentive, too.

I did continue having surgeries with the ear, nose and throat doctor. Changing doctors in the midst of a series of surgeries is tricky, like changing horses in midstream, and I think most doctors would be hesitant to climb in that saddle. For me, I felt enough confidence in the ear, nose and throat doctor to continue with him. Yet, if you believe your doctor is not doing a good enough job, make a change.

Finally, you need to be your own doctor. You need to keep on top of all procedures, medications, therapies, etc. Do not depend on your doctor or his office as your only source of care management. You need to know what is happening to you. You also need to ensure your general health is considered. Keep your primary care physician appraised of all procedures and any difficulties that may reflect on your general health. Be active in your healing process.

CHAPTER 2

Questions For Your Doctor

While you cannot prepare for an accident (excluding your grandmother's sage advice about underwear), non-emergency surgery allows for preparation and, as is often true, the more prepared the better.

This is embarrassing to admit. I went into my first cancer surgery with scarcely a clue what was going to happen. At the time, I convinced myself I was being brave. I wasn't going to let this new dilemma get to me. The accident had taken so much of my life away, I was not about to give the cancer a moment more than needed.

I decided to deal with my surgeries as they came, a swaggering, cavalier kind of valor. Looking back, I realize I was angry, frustrated and terrified. Yes, I'd been through it before and it was hell. I did not want another facial assault, so I closed my eyes and showed up at the dermatologist's office, letting his scalpel, like that baseball, bash into my life.

Dumb.

If you are going in for facial surgery, there are many things you need to know. Ask your doctor:

> "How do I care for myself after the surgery? (e.g., How often do I change my bandages? What medications will I take?) What are warning signs? When and how do I contact you?"

Specific instructions—that's what you need. Your doctor will give you written information addressing these issues. Be sure to go over these instructions and get your questions answered. I hope that you will have a caregiver and they, too, need to be informed.

I was not well informed after my first cancer surgeries. The written information I received covered little and when I asked about warning signs and "what if" scenarios I got a casual "don't worry about it—everything will be fine" reply.

I should have worried. Everything was not fine.

On Friday before Labor Day weekend, my flap down/skin rearrangement surgery, which took over four hours, was performed at a "day surgery" place. My doctor later agreed that was too long and intense a surgery for a day facility.

By Monday, Labor Day, I had uncontrollable vomiting and was unable to hold anything down, including my painkillers. We phoned my doctor's office. Living in a small town means we did not have a twenty-four-hour pharmacy so the physician's assistant suggested either my husband drive the hour and a half to his office to pick up suppositories that would stop my vomiting or I discontinue all liquid, food and medication and perhaps my vomiting would end. I recall a colorful array of language erupting from me upon receipt of his advice. Thankfully, our pharmacist (and friend), returned to town from vacation and I got the medication I needed.

What a nightmare and completely unnecessary.

Be informed of the things that can go wrong and how/when to contact your doctor. Have both painkillers AND nausea suppositories available after surgery. A lot of folks have trouble digesting painkillers. Make sure you have a backup to end vomiting.

Smartphones and email can be a great help. Infection is the greatest fear after surgery. Redness and swelling are signs of infection but they are also common in surgical areas. A few photos sent to your doctor can save time and worry.

"How bad am I going to look immediately after my surgery? How might my job be affected by my appearance? When can I go back to work?"

Concern over post-surgical appearance is not vanity; it is survival. Perhaps you will be one of the lucky ones. You will need little work and your change in appearance will be slight. On the other hand, you may end up like me.

Once the flap down and skin rearrangement surgery was complete, I looked diabolical. Even with a bandage covering much of my face, children would not come near me. Without a bandage, most men could not look at me. Women did better, but it took a stomach settling determination to gaze at me for long.

Yes, I was that bad.

My appearance was temporary, and remembering that helped get me through. My unquenchable and rather macabre sense of humor helped enormously also. Yet, there is no denying those first six weeks were arduous.

I live in a very small town—a modernized version of Mayberry. Thus, autonomy was impossible. Luckily, I did not work outside the home, so I could choose to avoid contact with others. For six weeks, I rarely left the house. I waited three weeks after my surgery to make my premier "to town" appearance. Lon Cheney never had a bigger entrance. Several people stepped back to get out of my way. Many gaped. One clerk looked at me, burst into tears and hugged me.

Months later, I asked my doctor's physician's assistant how long they recommended patients take time off work after a surgery like mine. She said one week, two if the person works in unclean conditions. Important piece of advice here—do not listen to this woman.

Do not automatically assume your doctor's advice is the best advice. The sad truth is, many doctors are more concerned with insurance companies and keeping your employer happy than they are with you. Even doctors, like mine, who sincerely care for their patients, often have limited knowledge of the healing process and accept insurance-company-driven policies (like getting back to work too soon) as acceptable.

Do not rush back to work before you are ready. Take the time you need even if you have to fight for it. Your body and mind require rest and good care. All of us know individuals who rushed back to work after injury or illness only to experience setbacks. In the end, they missed more work and cost themselves more money than if they had simply allowed themselves time to heal. Consider this; what is the best way to mend a sprained ankle—keep running on it or let it rest for a few days? Time to recover is time well spent.

Besides, your employer might not want you back right away.

Let's go back to that diabolical picture I painted of myself. Imagine me walking up to your table at a romantic little café and saying, "My name is Lois, and I will be your server."

Doesn't go over too well, does it?

A brutalized appearance does not work in many professions. If you are in one of these professions, you need to make plans with your employer about how to proceed. If you are a salesclerk, could you switch to inventory for the next six weeks? Could you move from public relations to advertising for a while?

Don't sell yourself short either. Employees who understand positions aside from their own make smarter workers. Remind your employer of that.

Another problem with getting right back to work is infection. Skin is highly susceptible to infection, especially the face, and you need to keep your skin clean and away from contagions.

What is your workplace like and what can you do to make it as germ-free as possible? Are you a physical laborer? This is not a good time to "pump up" and highly vacillate the skin or to expose your face to dirt and grime. Is light duty work available? Immediately after surgery is not when you want to catch a cold so avoid those cubicle coughers.

Be protective. Having gone through several infections, I can assure you infections are a pain in the butt at best and at worst, a serious disruption to the healing process.

"How long will it take my face to heal? What will I look like?"

When I initially approached my Tucson doctor about a third reconstruction, he would not schedule a consultation until a full year after my last surgery, thus, allowing my face to settle. Friends noticed differences in my face nearly two years after my final surgery in Tucson. It takes time to reach your end result. Part of this is the face settling in, a big part is learning to live with, work with and accept your facial differences.

Patience is required.

What will you look like in the end? Be prepared to hear this is a gray area. Plastic surgery is not an exact science. A nip here and tuck there do not necessarily add up as planned. After my accident, I was called into my doctor's office to choose what I wanted my nose to look like. While I was pleased with the work done, my nose did not look like what I chose.

How you look is not the exclusive domain of your surgeon's scalpel either. In the pages ahead, I include many techniques to maximize your appearance and you will undoubtedly discover more on you own. In addition, while I berate myself for not being better informed, there is another potential mistake you can make: knowing too much.

Thinking back to my accident, I believe if I had known from the beginning how much was ahead of me, I would have been overwhelmed. Instead, one surgery led to another surgery, then another. I was progressing up a ladder, not trying to reach the top in a single bound. It was not until a year after my accident that I realized the fatigue and memory loss I experienced were not caused by continual surgeries but by head injury.

In retrospect, I think I needed to first have my facial surgeries completed before thinking about living with head injury. Perhaps you are different. You might want every bit of information available from the beginning. Just be cautious of becoming overwhelmed.

CHAPTER 3

Getting ready for surgery

I hate preparing for surgery. It is a cold reminder of what is ahead. Yet, effort put in before surgery will make your post-op better. It is time well spent.

Preparing Your Body

Begin with your skin. It is about to go through an ordeal so help prepare it. Keep your skin clean and hydrated. Facials are an excellent idea. If your skin is dry, put effort into moisturizing. You want your skin as supple as possible.

The best things I've found for skin hydration are coconut oil and Shea butter combinations. A friend of mine makes a fabulous mix that includes mango and coconut butters. Look for local producers of lotions. It's amazing what folks come up with and often their product is fresh and without preservatives. Be careful of the products you put on your face, especially cleansers. Think gentle not stringent, simple rather than a long list of chemicals.

Don't forget to exfoliate. A washcloth can do the trick. Massaging your face is good for both muscles and circulation. The rule of thumb is stretch the skin, don't compress it. You can massage your face while watching TV or reading a book. It is a good habit to develop, especially just before sleep.

Have your teeth cleaned before surgery and if possible, any needed dental work completed. Not only will you gain a healthy mouth, an asset to healing, but also it is apt to be some time before you want a dentist stretching and contorting your mouth. However, do not have dental work done less than one week before surgery; it releases toxins.

It's time to get a haircut, and you may want a little shorter cut than usual to allow more time until your next appointment. If you are due for a perm or coloring, now is the time, but have both completed at least a week before surgery because both can irritate your skin. If you're considering a new look, this is a good time. Do not decide to forgo hair care. You are about to go through some lousy changes in your appearance. You'll be surprised how nice a good hair day feels.

Your whole body needs preparing, too. Good food, rest and exercise—these are always important but especially when preparing for surgery. A vitamin supplement paying special attention to C, B complex, iron and calcium is a good idea. An over-the-counter liquid equivalent to a vitamin B shot is now available. Taking the herb arnica can reduce swelling. Do not go into surgery constipated and be aware that painkillers can cause constipation. Have stool softeners and laxatives available.

Most doctors provide a long list of things to stop taking including aspirin and blood thinners, as well as many vitamins, herbs and minerals. I've watched this list grow exponentially, to the point I find it overly cautious, so instead of stopping fish oil, I reduced the amount I took. Know how you react. If you bleed easily, or if your surgery is extensive, take every precaution.

You may feel stressed and find your sleep disrupted. A bit of light exercise an hour or two before bed is helpful to me. An evening walk is ideal and provides that often prescribed fresh air. I have other ideas in the chapter ahead on sleep. If your sleep continues to be disrupted, consult your doctor. You need to be rested. It will enhance your healing process.

Preparing Your Home

You want your environment to be clean. In particular, scour your bathroom and make sure there are plenty of fresh towels and tissues. I am not a fan of antibacterial soap and all of my doctors during my final reconstruction recommended not using it. Soap and hot water are all you need. Freshly make your bed before surgery and run your pillows through the dryer to decrease dust. Have a change of sheets and several extra pillowcases ready, as you will want to change your linen often, pillowcases daily.

Getting your entire home spic and span is ideal though unnecessary, but do clean those places you will spend most of your time (e.g., your bed, your favorite recliner).

You will want an ice chest next to your bed with an ample supply of crushed ice for your face. If you have to crawl out of bed and down the hall to the fridge, you may forgo the effort. Icing after surgery is essential to minimize swelling. Your doctor may tell you to use your ice pack on and off. If your surgery is minor, that is good advice but for extensive surgery, I found enough heat is created for nearly continual icing.

You'll want fluids and a little food supply next to your bed because the kitchen may be too far away. Juice and a few crackers are not adequate. You'll need substantial food to take with your painkillers—applesauce, pudding, even jerky.

Don't forget yogurt with lactobacillus. It will help counter the ill effects of the antibiotics. Cranberry juice helps flush anesthesia from your system. Eating small amounts numerous times a day is easier on a post-op digestive track than full meals. I always make chicken soup before surgery. What illness or injury can't be helped by chicken soup?

Have things such as medications and bandages easily available. A special note to women: Your likelihood of getting a yeast infection is increased due to antibiotics and stress. Be prepared.

A Place to Stay Immediately After Surgery

I have a grievance against the American Medical Association. What is the first rule of first aid? Do not move the victim. Yet, as patients, we are run through day surgeries and pushed out the door so quickly my husband and I refer to the process as "slice and dump."

Follow the first aid advice when possible— stay put. If your surgery is in a hospital, you can stay up to twenty-four hours and still be considered outpatient care. Take advantage of the time, even if your doctor encourages you to leave. Make sure the nurses keep up with your ice.

For my first surgery in Tucson, which took over four hours, I opted to spend the night in the hospital—a personal cost of $700. I was tempted to forego the stay, but forced myself and my checkbook into it.

The stay was amazingly therapeutic. It was the right choice. If you are at a day surgery, you have no option but to leave, and it is my experience that you will be pushed out the door as quickly as possible.

Do not leave before urinating (watch for blood in the urine) or before you are able to move about comfortably. If you live some distance from the hospital, you should spend the night after surgery in a hotel nearby. Your doctor may insist on this because the first twenty-four hours is when hemorrhaging is most likely to occur.

Make the hotel aware of your surgery and when making the reservation, request that they give your room an extra-thorough cleaning. Once settled, try to move as little as possible. You will need mini versions of all things listed above for home use (e.g., ice chest, food).

Someone to Watch over You

You will need someone checking on you for at least the first forty-eight hours and beyond that someone nearby you can call in case of emergency. If you are unable to find someone, tell your doctor. Nursing services can be arranged, but planning is required.

I have heard far too many nightmare stories about people left alone after surgery. One friend of mine visited a woman two days after her retina reattachment surgery. The woman was barely conscious. The poor thing had had nothing but water for two days because she was too weak to go to the kitchen for food.

Be smarter than this.

Something to Look Forward To

This is the only part of preparing for surgery I like, thinking of things I would enjoy doing while recouping. For me, it is a stack of books; for you it may be a few movies or crossword puzzles. How about doing research for that trip to France you've dreamed of? All of us have things we want to do but can't find the time. You will be confined to quarters. Time is available.

Make sure you are planning enjoyable things, not preparing taxes or some other grueling task (unless you like preparing taxes). You will be going through some unpleasant days. Something to look forward to can make the time easier.

The Day of Surgery

Your doctor will tell you when you can have your last food and last liquid. I strongly recommend taking advantage of that time, even if you have to wake up in the night. The liquid in particular is important because you want to be as hydrated as possible. I drink cranberry juice that last hour. It helps flush anesthesia from your system and keeps your digestion healthy.

Take a long, hot shower just prior to leaving for the hospital. This is the only time I recommend anti-bacterial soap. Use it in your hair, too. Give your teeth a thorough cleaning and rinse with antiseptic mouthwash.

Be as relaxed as possible. I am notoriously late, but on days of surgery, I make sure to arrive early and unhurried. Remind yourself you've prepared for this day so there is no need to click through a mental list of what you might have forgotten to do. (Those things you did forget now fall into the "forget about it" category.) Choose music and conversation that relaxes you. Leave politics for another day.

Once admitted, make a conscious effort to withdraw into a relaxed state— prayers, meditation, deep breathing—whatever works for you. Some people watch television or chat idly but unless you need the distraction, I find it best to concentrate on relaxing in silence.

Your doctor, anesthesiologist and nurses will visit just prior to surgery. If you have special needs or concerns, voice them. For me, it is spiritual needs. Prior to surgery, I arranged to anoint my doctor's hands with holy oil. I have physical needs, too. I request an ice pack for my neck immediately after surgery to prevent headache.

Do not be shy about asking for such things. I've found doctors and staff to be not only helpful, but also appreciative of these things that are important to me.

Take ice with you if you will not be anesthetized. When I had my Mohs surgery to remove my cancer, I was not anesthetized and the doctor began by giving me shots in the face. They were horribly painful—and unnecessarily so. If you pack your face with ice just prior to a shot, your skin will be numb and you shouldn't experience pain. Some doctors are aware of this; others, like the doctor I saw, are not.

Do not take the chance. Take ice with you and ice pack your face just prior to a shot. In addition, during a checkup, your doctor may want to reduce your facial swelling by giving you cortisone shots in your face. (Some doctors oppose cortisone to the face.) These are also quite painful. Again, ice-pack your face.

CHAPTER 4

Caring for Yourself Immediately After Surgery

The first days after surgery set the pace for your healing process. It is a time to turn your thoughts inward and focus on healing.

Your doctor will probably recommend your surgical area should be left alone for the first day or two. Afterward, keep your incisions clean and well lubricated. Antibacterial ointment is typically no longer recommended and I think for good reason. If you are advised to use an antibacterial ointment, be cautious of its intensity.

I had a nasty reaction to a triple antibiotic cream. My skin became very irritated and my healing process was disturbed. If you are advised to use antibacterial ointment, have a gentler backup available, such as simple petroleum jelly.

My guru plastic surgeon in Tucson recommended that I put on my face only what could go into my eye. I had some healing difficulties after one of his surgeries. I did not follow this advice and overdid some home remedies. When I took his advice of gentler treatment and leaving the area alone, I fared better. Though it may seem unpleasant, let areas crust over rather than trying to continually wash them. If this condition embarrasses you, wear gauze over the affected area while around others.

In addition, if you tend to pick at scabs as I do, gauze will help keep you away. You will want to keep your entire face moisturized so have lotion on hand. Use a newly opened jar and wash your hands frequently because each time you dip in, you are potentially adding germs. Drink plenty of liquids to hydrate you and your skin.

Be aware of signs of infection and contact your doctor immediately if you suspect it. It is better to err on the side of caution. A few good quality digital pictures emailed to your doctor might save you a trip to his office.

Don't be a hero when it comes to pain. Men in particular have a hard time with this and let's face it, most of us despise the side effects of painkillers. Yet, like it or not, painkillers are needed after surgery, especially when the face is involved. Do not try going without or even cutting back on painkillers for the first few days. You may leave the hospital feeling quite pain-free. That euphoria of drugs and adrenalin may keep your pain away for a while, perhaps even until the next day.

Shortly after the surgery to eviscerate my eye, I felt surprisingly well, so my husband and I went out to breakfast. Seven hours later, I was in the worst pain I've ever experienced. No matter how well or euphoric you feel at first, eventually, the pain is going to hit. Be ready with a buffer of painkiller in your system. Keeping pain away is far easier than getting rid of it. Think of it this way; a fox locked out of the henhouse is one thing. Getting a fox out of the henhouse once he's inside is another.

Rest is your best medicine. When I was a teenager, I would quickly recoup from flu and colds by sleeping for hours on end. As adults, this process gets tougher, but it is still a good goal. When you are asleep, your body can fully concentrate on healing.

Sleep sitting up. Doing so prevents swelling. After my final surgery, a facelift with some revisions, the only swelling I had on my right side was when I slept flat. The first time was four days after surgery. I laid flat for just a few hours and the swelling was immediate.

The second time I swelled from lying flat was eleven days after surgery. I thought enough time had passed, but again I was swollen. Use plenty of pillows, give your neck good support and consider a disposable heat wrap on your shoulders to relax your muscles. (If using an electric heating pad, watch that it is not too hot and rotate on/off frequently.)

Watch for tension around your temples and jaw and massage those muscles frequently. If your neck gets achy or you develop headaches, icepack your neck. This will numb the pain and prevent swelling of your neck muscles. You can ice your neck and have heat on your shoulders at the same time. Experiment and find what works best for you. Make yourself as comfortable as possible.

You need good rest.

I mentioned a caregiver before, but it is important enough to reiterate that you need a caregiver, at least for the first few days. The caregiver should keep track of your medication, make sure you eat, help you get in and out of bed safely, etc.

If you must perform these tasks yourself, take every precaution. Do not rely on your memory for the first few days. Drugs and the trauma of surgery can make even the most astute mind foggy. Write things down (e.g., when and how much medication you take, when you last ate). Trying to keep a tally in your head can be stressful and disrupt your rest.

Instead, write things down and set an alarm to tell you when to take medications. Also, be cautious moving around. You may be unsteady and dizzy.

Perhaps most important: ICE.

As stated before, your doctor may suggest on and off icing but I find, if surgery is extensive, nearly continual icing is best. Don't forget to have a cooler with ice, as well as food, next to your bed. Steady snacking is preferred to meals.

Watch your blood pressure after surgery, especially if you tend toward high blood pressure. Mine shoots up a few days after surgery, the more extensive the surgery, the higher it goes. I suppose it's only natural. Though surgery is planned and sterile, it is no less an assault on your body than a car accident. Discuss with your doctor how high is too high and what you should do if your blood pressure reaches those heights.

Constipation commonly occurs after surgery, in part due to painkillers. Have stool softeners and suppositories available. Do not let constipation go unchecked. If needed, use polyethylene glycol powder, which is used to clean the colon before a colonoscopy. Be cautious, though. It is a powerful medication and can cause diarrhea.

CHAPTER 5

Greeting the Public after Surgery

The hardest thing I ever did was walk into our valley's City Market after my second cancer surgery. I looked horrible and people reacted accordingly. If ever a soldier deserved a badge for courage, it was me that day.

Sometimes, I cry remembering it, not only from the experience, but also out of sympathy for that woman who I was. I won't sugarcoat this. If you are going through the kind of surgeries I did, you have some tough days ahead. Over and over, my face was sliced. Time and again, I faced the public. Yet, I survived, in part because I learned to deal with public viewings on my own terms.

Long after my third cancer surgery, I wore a bandage on my face in public, and prior to that surgery, nonstop after my cancer removal. I reiterate, I looked awful. I did not want to share my looks with the public so I determined what part of my face was available for viewing.

Share your face with others when you are ready. This includes your kind but curious neighbor who stops by to get a peek at you. It is inevitable; a disfigured face attracts attention. Plus, the face is fair game, at least in our part of the world. No one approaches a woman who has had a mastectomy and says, "Could you lift your shirt? I want to see what they did to you." Yet, my face was often scrutinized and commented upon.

The attention felt between uncomfortable and exasperating. By covering up, I was better able to choose when, where, and with whom I shared my face. It gave me a sense of control at a time when much of my life was out of my control.

Before I go on, I want to make one thing clear. Staying home, refusing to see others or more accurately, refusing to let them see you, is not an answer. Isolation leads to depression. There is nothing about you that should be isolated and do not feel ashamed of your appearance.

The reason I prepared my face with bandages before going out in public was not because my looks were shameful, but because I wanted to curb people's reactions to me. It may be a subtle difference, but it is an important one.

Your appearance is not a disgrace.

Nothing about you needs hiding. The reason I urge you to consider bandages is they allow you to choose how and when to share your appearance and to help soften responses to you.

Instead of fretting and hoping no one noticed me, before going out, I would steel myself. People were going to notice me and I accepted this with as much kindness and understanding as I could muster. I suggest you do the same.

Let's say you are three weeks off surgery; your face is brutalized and you have a bandage in place. You are at the grocery store and a man walks toward you. He looks at you. He looks again. Now, he realizes he is staring. He is embarrassed.

The best response to him is to smile, nothing fancy, just a simple smile. It is a way of saying, "It's okay that you noticed."

A reassuring smile puts others at ease, allowing you to feel at ease also. Only once did a woman get close to my face, glaring into my left eye with the intensity of a collector. It was awful; yet, she was the pathetic one, not me.

Before going out, take a discerning look at your face. How much do you want to cover and how much are you willing to release to public view? Your first response may be wanting to wrap yourself like a mummy. Look again. You are not going to appear "normal" but in most cases, there are only a few areas severe enough to warrant covering.

Time for the gauze pads and scissors. Cut a bandage to cover as small an area as possible. Now look again. Chances are there is more Band-Aid to snip away. Bandages don't have to be angulated either. Customize both shape and size to suit your needs. When you get a design you like, make several so you always have one on hand.

In October of 2010, my left eye was eviscerated. I had to wait six weeks before being fitted with a prosthetic eye. Eleven days after surgery, I dressed as a pirate for Halloween, not your run of the mill pirate, either. Short skirt, low cut blouse, gorgeous red, head scarf shimmering; I looked like a contestant in a Betty Grable lookalike contest.

My eye patch was standard black with an elastic band wrapped around my head. While the patch worked well for Halloween, I did not want it for daily use. Instead, I took my least favorite pair of glasses and covered the left lens. Those became my around the house glasses. I felt I needed better coverage in public though.

The bandages I found for eyes were gleaming white and big, not what I wanted. Instead, I took a piece of flesh tone Ace bandage and cut it more or less into an eye shape.

It still was not right.

I looked like I had solid flesh over my socket, which was almost as unnerving as no eye. I then took white tape and edged the patch with it, a finished product. The patch was small, fitting almost completely behind my glasses. The color blended with my face yet with the white edging, it looked like a patch. Clear tape held it in place, and I was off.

I share this mundane eye patch information for two reasons. First, snipping away at bandages gets you actively involved. You are not a victim of circumstance, but rather, making decisions about your appearance. It is a way of gaining some control.

Second, customizing bandages gets you acquainted with your face. There is a tendency after facial trauma not to want to see how you look; yet, learning to accept and work with your appearance is important to healing. When I worked to look my best, it helped me accept my facial challenges. I gained confidence in greeting the public, too.

CHAPTER 6

Healing

The road to healing can be traveled many ways. You can jump back into life, ignoring your healing process as much as possible and, somehow, the magnificent machine you call your body will repair itself. You can put a little effort in, even give occasional thought to your predicament, but in general push on and, again, your body will eventually persevere.

The road I recommend is quite different: Jump in, both feet first.

As our dear Catholic priest, Father Bill Nelson quoted Emerson: "Life is not a destination; it is a journey." Like it or not, you are now on a journey of healing. It is a journey of body, mind and soul. Open your eyes. Take a look around.

DO NOT keep busy. DO think about what is happening.

In American society, and much of the world, we have become so busy we digressed from contemplation. There was a time when old codgers sitting in porch rockers were considered wise, in part because they had seen much of life, but it was also because they sat, rocked and thought. They contemplated the past, the future and all points in between.

Never underestimate the power of thought.

With concentrated thought, you can help your body repair itself. You can delve deep into yourself and find strength you may not know existed. The deeper you go, the more you grow as a person. "Man's mind, stretched with a new idea, never returns to the same dimensions," Einstein once said.

For those of us repairing battered faces, healing is not simply an idea but a disruption of life. There is much to learn, much to be gained. Don't go through this journey blinded by busyness. Take time to think, and to process, what is happening to you.

Your doctors and your family will probably give the opposite advice. Got a problem? Keep busy. Worried? Don't think about it. I respectfully disagree.

If you are healing, (and if you are not, it is still good advice) take time to relax and ponder. Let your mind wander through thought. Not every day thoughts of job and family, but the big questions, "Why am I here?" "What is this thing called life about?" These are the thoughts I mean. I don't care if you are Catholic, agnostic, or expecting UFOs to land, this is a time to think about life—the big picture. To me, it is soul time.

As I mentioned, my life was quite different when my accident occurred than when I was diagnosed with cancer. In 1996, that baseball knocked me out of an active life. I was involved in the business my husband and I owned, an aspiring author and a very active mom.

I think my husband and son felt a hole gouged out of their lives after my accident, but to me it was a gaping fathom. Yet, despite that feeling, I took time to think; about what had happened to me, about what it meant. I prayed. I did a lot of journaling. I spoke with friends. I thought about life, what it all meant, and it became a part of my healing process.

When my cancer was diagnosed in 2006, I was already living a more contemplative life. Though I was deeply hurt when I learned I had cancer, (also scared, frustrated and downright pissed off), in my heart, I knew nothing happened without opportunity to grow. I knew that each occurrence in life had meaning, even this stupid, unfair, horrible cancer, and it could work to my betterment.

I was ready, at least in part, to spend time in my own head and heal.

Good thing. After my initial surgeries, I was thoroughly knocked down. I've described my brutalized appearance. I felt as good as I looked. Between the minimal sight in my left eye and the now protruding "Ferengi butthead" which blocked my peripheral vision, I was prevented from driving.

We live several miles from town so for seven weeks I spent much of my time at home. Add to that my "terrify small children" appearance and my confinement to quarters seemed appropriate. I sat. I prayed. I thought.

I cannot encourage you enough; explore your spirituality. It is a wonderful tool for healing. Not interested in spirituality? Then explore the essence of your being, delve into your yin and yang, whatever it is you do to go deep into yourself. Your soul (or whatever term you use) holds the essence of you.

Failing to connect your soul to your healing process is a void that cannot otherwise be filled. I think of the paintings of farm scenes done in the 1500s by Pieter Brueghel the Elder. Pastoral scenes depicted workers as mindless, animal-like laborers. As they plodded through their chores, they appeared void of thought, even feeling. The sophistication of computers and college educations do not prevent us from being the same brute laborers.

When we mediate and nurture our souls, we fully connect with ourselves, and from this, we can heal. You will probably find yourself in a position of inactivity anyway. Take advantage of it. Sit down in a rocker, clear your mind of thought and gently rock. Take your thoughts deep. I find when I delve into deep thought, I am truly living the moment. Things feel a little different, a bit more real. There is simplicity and peace, yet, energy as well.

What will you experience? I don't know. Take the time to find out.

Once you reach a centered state of mind, you may, as I often do, find insight. I can look more clearly at what has happened to me and where I need to go with my healing. When I sense the depth of my soul, I breathe deeply, using the beauty of my soul to soothe and heal.

Am I losing you? Does this sound too "out there"?

Let's try a more practical analogy. Let's say you are boarding one of those super colossal roller coasters; the kind that drop one hundred sixty degrees, twist upside down, then rocket upward. As you board with the screaming crazies, you snuggle into your seat in a padded rubber suit, blindfold and a headset playing soothing music.

Why are you so attired?

Because you plan to feel nothing, see nothing and hear nothing of the adventure you are about to undergo. Much like Brueghel's farm laborers, you have decided on business as usual. Yet, does it make sense to enter such an adventure and ignore it?

I don't think so. Then why should you go through something as traumatic as cancer or a catastrophic accident/illness—whatever has brought you to this point—and then try to live life in the shallow depths of "as usual"?

Let's look at the man on the roller coaster again, all bundled up and trying to keep his mind off what is happening to him. I don't think it will work. In fact, I think it will backfire. By not facing the adventure at hand, his imagination has opportunity to step in and create a ride more frightening than reality.

Live the moment. Spend time in contemplation and look to your soul for help. It is the best route for the healing journey.

There is a difference between contemplation and self-absorption. Depression, self-absorption at its worst, is a threat to anyone going through the healing process. Undoubtedly, that is why the advice to keep busy and ignore illness or injury is given. Busyness can be a means of warding off depression, though not a good one, in my opinion.

Remember, spending time in contemplation concentrating on the healing process is different from obsessing about the unfairness of getting cancer or the fear of always looking like a monster.

Anger and anxiety will emerge. These feelings need to be acknowledged. Yet, anger and anxiety should not be permitted to take over. When a wave of anger hits, accept it. Let it work its way through you, even scream about it, but keep it moving. Do not ruminate on this negativity. Give frustration and fear voice, but not center stage.

"Healing Process."

Remember those two words. You are healing. You are in a process. Work to make it an active, positive state of being, and delve deep into yourself. There was a time the unexamined life was considered less than life. I think that theory still holds true. Sit. Think. It will do you good.

THE HEALING PROCESS

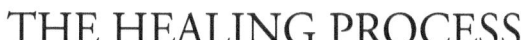

CHAPTER 7

The Odyssey Begins

You are feeling almost human again. The healing journey has begun. Where do you go from here?

My best advice: Take it slow. Be patient. Initially, you may find, as I did, that how you feel is so varied and unpredictable that planning is difficult. If possible, begin your journey on a daily basis.

It was during my initial cancer surgeries that I began my coffee ritual. Rather than setting the alarm for the last possible moment to arise, I began getting up early. I would make a cup of coffee and settle into my rocker by the window. I would sit and rock, watching light pierce the darkness. I would let my mind wander the depths I mentioned in the previous chapter; my purpose in life, the meaning of life itself. I would plan my day.

It is time to belly up to the mirror, too. If you have been following my advice, (surely) you are already working with your face. Now is the time to gaze deeper.

It isn't an easy task. After my initial cancer surgeries, I remember wondering if Lois was even there anymore. It was an eerie, unsettling feeling; like being dropped into a Twilight Zone episode. I think if the lack of recognition had continued for a longer period, it could have damaged my personality. After all, self-recognition is essential to a baby's development; how can it be any less important to an adult?

Fortunately, I recognized my right eye. Beneath the twisted, battered skin, Lois was looking back at me.

That piece of self- recognition became the stone upon which to build my new face. I realized it would be a new face, too. I had already been through reconstruction after my accident and, given the degree of damage done in post-cancer surgeries, I had no doubt that a long road was ahead. Me looking back at me created a bond upon which to build. Piece by piece, I was determined to lose deformity and create the best face possible.

There are immediate, practical reasons for getting acquainted with your face as well. I had infection and deterioration after the second cancer surgery. By being familiar with my face, I noticed the signs of trouble. Another consideration is that you will be interacting with others: friends and family, clerks in the store where you shop.

Familiarity will help you feel more comfortable with your looks. The more comfortable you feel, the easier it is for others to accept them. This is also the time to set goals for your looks. Be an active participant in your development, both by interacting with your doctor and working toward improvement on your own.

Learn to look with love at your new face, no matter how frightening your appearance. Stir your compassion. Think of your face as a child who has fallen from her bike. She is muddy, bloody and her face is wet with tears and a runny nose; yet, she still needs to be taken into your arms.

A top no-no in my book is referring to any part of your body as "bad." There is nothing bad in your body, or mine. As my son's principal used to say, "It's all good." Labeling a healing area bad is counterproductive. If you want to hinder a child's development, start calling him the bad boy. Predictably, he will withdraw, fail to thrive, and probably become a mean little bugger. Is the body any different?

When I referred to my odd looking, mostly-blind eye, I came up with several scenarios. My favorite was "I have a natural eye (my right) and an artist's rendition of an eye (my left)." If others, particularly doctors, referred to my eye as bad, I gently but firmly corrected them. My eye functioned with less efficiency than it once did and it needed extra care. That was not bad, just reality.

Appreciate your body's amazing ability to heal. Don't reprimand it for falling short of perfection.

Along with a slow, nurturing launch to your healing journey, keep this in mind: The healing process is a tango, not a forward march. You will feel better, look better, then suddenly be spun backward, your face swollen anew. You will overdo and bring on problems. You will laze too long and feel set back. There will be times that, for no apparent reason, you slip backward.

It is all part of the healing process. Spin, dip, twirl back, press forward; this is the rhythm of healing. Leave marching to the halftime band. Dance the tango of your healing and be confident that you will cross the floor.

CHAPTER 8

Dealing with Pain

The first few days after surgery, it is important you take prescription painkillers regularly. After a few days, I am generally able to wean off them.

How do I judge whether I need prescription painkillers?

First, can I sleep? I need to be able to get to sleep and, if I wake up, go back to sleep. If pain is keeping me from doing so, I take medication. Second, am I able to concentrate and function? Some disruption in my day from pain is acceptable, but if I am constantly disrupted, that is too much. Last, am I able to put a smile on my face? If pain is so dire that I am oppressed by it, I take medication.

Pain is a strange thing. Just the word can make us cringe. Yet, the truth is, pain is an important part of the body's defense. Pain is the alarm that tells us something is wrong. By learning to listen to pain, we can help solve the problem.

Skin, particularly on the face, is susceptible to infection and other problems. Pain is often the first alert there is trouble, so listen closely to the message.

Basically, pain comes in three types. There is normal/acceptable pain. This is the everyday garden variety of scratchy pain from stitches, aches of bruised muscles and if you have nerve damage as I do, occasional "shooter" pains that feel like shots of electricity. These are of no concern.

Next is a gray area, new pain that shows up days after surgery or pain that was there before but has intensified. There are a lot of reasons for gray area pain, most are of no concern; yet, your body has set off an alarm. Pay attention.

Then there is abnormal/unacceptable pain. Severe pain, intense pain that feels hot or acute pain associated with nausea are all indications that it is time to get to the doctor.

My first response to pain is ice. I used to suffer from migraines. By lying down with an ice pack on my neck at the first signs of a migraine, I could often avoid them. Ice reduces swelling that contributes to pain, and ice can numb pain.

Itching is another problem ice can solve. During my skin rearrangement surgery, I was literally scalped in order to move the skin on my forehead and scalp. Nerves were severed and as they regenerated, the itching was unbelievable. To this day, I have to be cautious of rubbing my forehead and scalp because too much stimulation can cause an itching frenzy.

Ice is my best relief; numbing and, thus, shutting off the itching.

A few years before my evisceration, I had terrible pain in my eye. Immediately, I put an ice pack next to, and for brief periods, on my closed eyelid. I then settled into a comfortable chair and tried to relax. I listened very closely to the pain, trying to discern its epicenter.

When pain is intense, it's difficult to track and sometimes it cannot be tracked. All of my eye hurt— front, back, inside, outside, even my lid. Yet, as I concentrated on the pain, it became more defined. I determined the epicenter was around the pupil. I locked my mind into that place, that pain. I tried to calm it. I took slow, soothing breaths.

Breathing techniques are great for pain relief, and I believe they should be in everyone's first aid kit. Lamaze for childbirth probably has the best breathing techniques. Yoga is another source.

Throughout our lives there are times we are overwhelmed by pain, both physical and mental. Knowing how to soothe body and mind through breathing is a great asset.

Often, I can get enough pain relief through ice, breathing, and concentration to allow myself to briefly fall into a sleep state akin to hypnosis. If I can reach that state, the pain alarm in my brain has a chance to turn off or at least lighten up.

Unfortunately, none of my techniques worked that day for my eye. The pain was severe and continued at full speed. For the second time in my life, I headed to the emergency room.

You may wonder why I mention this incident, as it appears to be a failure in my pain control techniques. Actually, it demonstrates my success. Ice, breathing techniques, tracking and then concentrating on soothing the pain and finally, dropping into a relaxed state, this is how I control pain. When I was unable to use that control, even in part, I knew I needed medical attention.

The problem was a severely irritated cornea. Removing eyelashes that were growing into my eye as well as medication eased the problem.

Understanding pain can help you control it. You cut your finger and pain comes from the cut—not really. You cut your finger and pain comes from your brain. Nerves at the cut have rushed a message to your brain that there's a problem and your brain sets off the alarm. Thank God it does, or you would leave your hand on a hot burner. Keep this process in mind when trying to soothe your pain.

First, try to discern the pain's source. I'm a big fan of massage and it isn't just for the relaxation. Massage heightens awareness of your body. My massage therapist's deft hands have taught me to find specific places on my body that are flared so instead of mass muscle discomfort, I can feel the exact spots that are problems.

Do the same in finding your pain. Sit back and listen to the pain. Track it with your mind to find the epicenter. Once found, consider if there is anything that would alleviate the pain. Back to the cut: does it need moisturizer, a new bandage or, if appropriate, ice?

Once you are sure everything possible has been done, relax and concentrate on soothing the pain. Send assuring thoughts that care has been administered and there is no longer need for the alarm. Soothe your pain as you would soothe a child with a skinned knee.

After injury or surgery, it is natural to protect the affected area. If you sprain your wrist, you will instinctively cradle your arm. This reaction is good, yet, can cause trouble. After having my eye eviscerated, I had a tendency to squint. In fact, I squinted so hard that I gritted my teeth. I was unaware I was doing this until some nasty headaches appeared via TMJ.

Massage, concentrating on not squinting and sending soothing thoughts that the trauma to my eye was over, brought an end to the problem.

Examine your posture after injury or surgery, keeping in mind your instinct to protect affected areas. Are your shoulders back or are you slouching? Is your head held straight or are you leaning it slightly down and to the right, protecting your injured jaw? Work to get your body in good alignment.

I am blind on my left side and I have a tendency to turn my head slightly to the left. Doing so provides some peripheral vision on my blind side. Unfortunately, tilting my head to the side, even slightly, can throw off my alignment. Keeping active, stretching, and massage all help. An excellent source is the book Pain Free by Pete Egoscue.

I had near miraculous results for both my neck and knee from the Pain Free program. I cannot recommend it highly enough. Also, for anyone healing the face, watch for tension at the edge of your jaw just below your ear, a place where many headaches begin. Massage and a warm pack can help.

After surgery, your face is apt to be quite swollen. A trick I learned was to soak my face in an Epsom salt bath. I would fill a large bowl with warm water and Epsom salt, then dunk my face, breathing out slowly to create soothing bubbles. However, do not wet unhealed skin. I made the mistake of using this technique too soon after my final surgery. My skin dried out and the suture line pulled apart, making healing difficult.

While the techniques I've discussed may not make you pain-free, they are valuable assets in pain relief. Consider acupuncture and hypnosis as well. You may wish to use over-the-counter painkillers. I strongly recommend avoiding Ibuprofen, Tylenol and other variations of acetaminophen. My husband had a horrible allergic reaction to acetaminophen, which left his extremities swollen and his skin peeling. I have since learned this is not a rare reaction.

If you do use these drugs, use them cautiously. Over-medicating with them can cause liver damage. Check the expiration date, too. Acetaminophen can cause liver damage if taken after it expires. Do not be lulled into thinking that because these are over-the-counter drugs, they are not potentially dangerous.

A final note on pain relief: Most of us enjoy occasional sympathy and giving a show and tell of wounds is a good way to get it. Yet, be warned that sharing the horrors of your pain may seem interesting subject matter, but in the telling, you are encouraging your mind to relive the memory. As discussed earlier, pain comes from the brain. By recalling pain, you can turn that pain on again. For example, you may feel a twinge of pain in your knee while telling about your skiing accident.

Leave memories of pain in the past. Keep to the sunny side of life—it's warmer.

CHAPTER 9

Exercise For Health and Healing

I have always exercised. Not that I'm a fanatic, or even in particularly good shape, but exercise has always been a part of my life. If it isn't a part or yours, it is time to rethink the subject. As the old adage goes, find something you enjoy doing, and when healing, find something that promotes your healing process.

For me, it was hula, the dance of the Hawaiian Islands. I love dancing, and I have taken classes in various forms. Hula was an easy addition and it can be very gentle, which is ideal when beginning exercise after surgery.

It is inadvisable to get your heart pounding soon after facial reconstruction. Doing so can promote swelling and irritate newly sutured areas. Plus, your energy needs to go to healing, not strenuous activity. Whatever exercise you choose, in the beginning, don't raise your blood pressure very much.

Concentrate on stretching and mild strengthening rather than aerobic workout.

Hula's most compelling attribute for me was its allure. Body swaying gently, hands telling a hypnotic tale, it is a beautiful dance and beauty was just what I needed, both after my accident and cancer reconstruction. As I danced the hula, I concentrated on making my movements as graceful as possible.

I tried to project beauty. As I danced, I envisioned my battered face becoming part of that beauty. Dancing the hula always brought a smile, sometimes cleansing tears as well.

There is another asset to hula, perhaps to all dance and activities such as yoga and tai chi, too. They encourage body harmony. Via their movements, there is concentration on moving parts of the body independently, yet, an awareness of the whole body. They synchronize you.

After my accident, I was battered and blinded in one eye. I felt out of sync. To help, I sat and moved my hands in unison, working to regain the oneness of my body.

Walking is another activity that allows you to choose your pace. Prior to my baseball accident, I was playing racquetball weekly. My first exercise after my accident was walking to the top of my drive and back, a one hundred twenty foot journey. It was a grueling trek, and I remember feeling proud of myself.

No matter what level of fitness you are coming from, take pride in your accomplishments. Whenever possible, walk outside, not on a treadmill. Leave the iPod at home. Instead, listen to, and become absorbed in, the world around you. Even if your turf is a chaotic city neighborhood, tune in. Live the moment. Let your walk become time to connect with yourself and the world around you.

In all outdoor activities, do not forget your hat. A baseball cap is not enough. I wear a big-brimmed gardening hat whenever I go outside and I keep it by the front door so I don't forget it. Wear sunscreen as advised but do not put it on newly sutured areas because it may cause irritation. Consider using zinc oxide. It is an excellent sunblock and good for your skin. Since hats do not protect you against reflective light and your sunscreen use may be limited, the best decision is to limit your time in the sun, especially in the beginning.

Refrain from most sports. Do not take the risk of being hit in the face. It's Murphy's Law. If ever you are going to take a blow to the face during a sport, it will happen after facial surgery. Think how foolish and painful a botched tennis return would seem if it meant another surgery to re-repair your nose.

In the beginning, make tennis and other such activities spectator sports. Swimming is great exercise, but check with your doctor before heading to the pool. In general, pool water is not recommended after surgery, but salt water is fine.

CHAPTER 10

Sleep

While preparing this chapter, I realized something odd. We train for physical fitness, even hire personal trainers; yet, we expect sleep to come naturally, without thought or effort. For many of us, sleep does not come easily. Instead, we toss, turn, and wander through some days half-awake. Yet, good sleep, like good physical fitness, can be improved with training.

The first question in sleep training is:

Are you allowing enough hours for sleep?

Sleep is one of the most individualized things we do, beginning with how much we need. Anywhere from six to ten hours is recommended, depending on the individual. That's a vast difference.

If you are unsure how many hours of sleep you need, begin with eight hours and note your reaction. If you wake up earlier than needed, try seven hours. Hone in on a consistent number. Having a consistent bedtime is just as important, researchers say. If each night you go to bed at 11:00, your body learns that 11:00 is the time to shut down. Set a time for bed and stick with it. While establishing your bedtime, even weekends should adhere to your rule.

Do not allow yourself to "cheat" until your sleep hours have become a habit. Even after they are established, make your late nights few. DVRs can record movies; good books are still in print the next day. Be strict with bedtime hours.

Evaluate your sleeping environment. A dark, cool, and quiet bedroom is optimal. In fact, in surveying my friends, I found the number one component of good sleep was a cool to cold room.

Your bed should be as comfortable as possible. Morning backache is a sign your bed is not firm enough. Waking up often to change sleeping positions may mean your bed is too hard. If your pillow needs several adjustments a night, buy another pillow, and keep searching until you find the right one. Fresh, soft linens add to a pleasant environment.

Another good rule: beds are for sleep and sex only. Beds are not for watching TV, reading, or checking Facebook. Those activities encourage wakefulness and the light they emit can disrupt a hormone that helps you sleep. Leave the bedroom for sleep and sex—period.

Develop a ritual as a prelude to sleep. After climbing into bed, I spend a moment massaging my face. Between the eyebrows and at the jaw are particularly susceptible to tension and be aware that tightness on the brows can indicate worry and at the jaw, anger. I massage lotion on my feet. A few deep breaths and I begin a prayer. Rarely do I not fall right to sleep.

Staying asleep is another matter. Often, two to four hours later, I am awake. I used to find this frustrating, which only added a sharper edge to my wakefulness. Now, if I wake up, I try to enjoy the luxury of rest. Life gets hectic. Who has time to lie and do nothing? For that matter, who would want to?

Night is different.

At night, I can lie in bed and let time roll by. It's what I'm supposed to do. I love my bed—soft and comfy. I like listening to the quiet of the night. I like the smell of lotion on my hands. I rub my feet together, enjoying the softness. Often, this bit of cuddling is enough to see me back to sleep.

If not, I tell myself stories, just as I did when I was a child. They are pleasant bits of dreamy make believe that bring a smile—as simple as hugging a missed friend, as complicated as heroically returning a woman's lost purse. They are the kind of stories that bring a bit of pleasure, but not excitement.

My goal is to return to sleep, and if I am lucky, that pleasant feeling will follow me into my dreams.

Some nights I wake up angry or worried; yet, I still try to react the same way. I look for simple pleasures; touch and smell are particularly important. Storytelling can occupy my mind, thus, blocking out other thoughts. Yet, sometimes these techniques are not enough.

I hate to admit it, but often politics is the culprit that steals my sleep. Some news report or debated issue can rile me. If I awaken upset by an issue, I try to turn my mind to prayers for peace, not just for "my side" or myself but for all. Peace becomes my focus, much like a mantra, and peace can soothe me back to sleep.

Sometimes, personal concerns rob my sleep. At night, worry can run through my mind like wildfire. If prayers for peace do not stop my worry, I then ask myself, "What can I do?" I require an immediate, simple, doable answer.

Let's say my worries come from a financial concern. "Did I make the payment? Was there enough money in our account? What if there isn't enough money?" I resolve that as soon as I arise, I will confirm the check was written and at eight o'clock sharp, call the bank to verify the check cleared. If problems remain beyond that, I will deal with them in the morning—a simple, doable solution.

I then demand the issue be closed. If worry returns to my thoughts, I quickly restate my resolve to (a) confirm the check and (b) call the bank and then demand the issue be closed. "But what if…" my worry tempts.

"No," I respond, issue resolved and discussion closed. By making my response firm, the issue is pushed away, and by developing a habit of dealing with nighttime concerns in a like manner, my sleep is rarely disrupted for long.

Without discipline, the mind near sleep can become a running wheel of what I call circle thought. In her elder years, dear Aunt Rose was often a victim of it. She would start a story, get nearly to the end, then start the telling all over again. At the edge of sleep, it is easy to get caught in circle thought, which is why a strong response is needed. Be firm, much like a parent to a child.

One friend of mine said she would worry about forgetting her solution. She suggested having a pen and paper by the bed to jot down the idea. If a quick notation brings peace, that is fine, but do not become a midnight stenographer.

Worry about others can steal my sleep. If my prayers for peace don't prevail, I try to step back from my concern. Too often, my worry for others has them frozen in a bad situation instead of thinking of them in the fluidity of life. My worry focuses only on what my loved ones are up against and what they might lack. I block the reality of their, and life's, resilience.

To soothe my concern, I remind myself that the struggles and failures of life are often our greatest building blocks. I try to envision my loved ones moving through their difficulties, not caught by them. I may even decide a simple, doable step to help. I remind myself to have faith in them, and in life.

Sometimes, relationships become so toxic that we need to step away. Though I loved a member of my family deeply and felt a real obligation via that love, I could not have her in my life, not directly. I did not feel safe around her and I had a young son to consider.

I cut the relationship to bare bones. Yet, severing our relationship felt wrong, bringing me sadness, concern for her, and many sleepless nights. I found solace through small acts of kindness to others in a similar circumstance. I felt that by helping a stranger, perhaps my family member would gain kindness from a stranger, too.

I see life this way; like a pond that we cast our words and actions into, creating ripples that, whether for good or ill, resonate back. Assuring myself that I was, at least, doing something, helped ease my sleeplessness. The good news is my family member's life became better and our relationship was restored.

There is another way to find peace for good sleep; I call it rocketing into the stratosphere. Take your mind away from the everyday and allow the lofty heights of the stratosphere to show you the forest instead of the chaos of trees. With distance, you see the past blending into itself, the present in motion, and the future full of possibilities.

Patterns in our life repeat again and again; yet, change is the only constant. It is a bit like the old soap operas; if you watched them every day, you were caught up in the whirlwind of intrigue. Yet, if you stepped away for a month then returned, little had changed. Sleep is often lost in the details. The stratosphere helps blur the edges.

While in the stratosphere, look at your past. If you are like me, some months ago, anger and worry were claiming your sleep. You were in a situation that would not resolve, at least not without a catastrophic outcome.

Time has gone by. Do you even remember what was so upsetting? Perhaps there were catastrophic results, but the planet is still twirling. If you look further back, there may be other such incidents. Remembering how quickly problems flare then resolve may help you face new worries with less alarm and more sleep.

Before coming down from the stratosphere, consider this: All things work for the greater good. "Good? How can you say that? Look at all the terrible things that happen: murders, famine, war. How can any of that be good?"

It is not the murder that is good, but life's response to it; a turn toward comfort, solace, even forgiveness. Famines devastate, but life turns to the good of renewal. War kills and destroys. We may someday destroy the planet in our fury; yet, in those final moments, life will be turning toward the greater good, trying to heal and soothe.

This is not a concept unique to me. Moving ever toward the greater good is the teaching of most religions. It is the basis of evolution. Belief in moving to the greater good may seem a lofty subject for the stratosphere; yet, it can also be a soothing remembrance amid life's complications. Everything must change.

Good is ever-present.

Be careful not to train yourself to wake up at night. Don't give yourself tasks, or even worse, rewards, for wakefulness. I used to have a series of prayers that I liked saying if I awoke. Eventually, I realized my anticipated enjoyment was waking me.

Getting up for a midnight snack can be a soothing break from restlessness, but it can also become a nightly habit. Repetition is the best way to train the mind. Make sure you are repeating good sleep habits.

While writing this chapter, I spent a lot of time observing my sleep patterns. At one point, I had a nasty cold that made sleep particularly difficult. The techniques I mentioned above were not helpful. It was not my mind that needed soothing, but my body.

I tried a technique more akin to hypnosis. I envisioned myself looking into a large, round bowl and having it close enough that all I could see was the inside of the bowl. The sides were uneven, a textured look, yet smooth. The color, an earthy, dark copper-brown. The bowl had no reflection nor was it absorbent, a blank slate.

I allowed nothing in the bowl. If a thought entered my mind, I envisioned the thought becoming a black and white photo, stopped without animation, and let it float away from the bowl.

My body became relaxed; aches, and pains eased. I concentrated only on the soothing earthen walls. I was able to hit the main breaker in my mind. No circuitry was running except my connection to the bowl. When I stopped concentrating on it, I was relaxed and near sleep.

I have been hypnotized on a few occasions, so my mind knew the level of disconnection I wanted to attain. I highly recommend a few sessions of hypnosis. Training your mind to drop into deep relaxation and disconnection is a great benefit, and not just for sleep. Throughout our lives, we experience times of extreme pain and/or anxiety.

Being able to disconnect and drop into relaxation, even in part, is a great asset.

Last year, I went through a period of unusual fatigue even though I was getting enough hours of sleep. My doctor was concerned that I was developing sleep apnea. I closely watched my sleep patterns and realized I was waking up overheated. I started Chinese medicines that eased the problem and I put a small fan beside my bed. The fan eased my overheating and if sleep apnea was a problem, the moving air made me breath deeper, eliminating that concern as well.

Diet should be considered when examining sleep. Sugar and caffeine are obvious thieves of good rest, but your unique system may have other things that bother you. My Italian husband makes fabulous spaghetti sauce, but tomatoes can mean I awaken with heartburn. Antacids before sleep usually do the trick. Also, look for foods that help you sleep. Two hours after a turkey dinner, I can hardly keep my eyes open.

There are external deterrents to good sleep as well. For me, it was my husband's snoring. I used to try turning him, but all that did was disrupt his sleep and frustrate me. One night, it occurred to me that his snoring was much like the olden days when the town crier walked the streets shouting, "Four o'clock and all's well!"

The crier undoubtedly awakened people, but I doubt that many complained. His proclamation told them they were safe. Now, when I awaken to my husband's snoring, I remind myself that we are safe in our bed, that we are together and at peace.

Odd as it seems, his snoring can be a comfort to me. But my husband is not a loud snorer—loud snoring can be a sign of health issues and should be investigated.

Work to minimize disruptions to your sleep environment, but be flexible. Becoming upset by noise or lights that you have no control over only adds to your fitfulness. As is often true in life, change the things you can and accept the things you cannot.

Any discussion of my sleep needs to include Fudd. Fudd is a worn stuffed animal my son gave me years ago. I sleep with Fudd every night. If I'm sad, I hug him. I travel with him. My friends know him. Am I crazy? Like a fox.

Pavlov's dogs have nothing on me. My reaction to Fudd is strong and immediate, comfort and relaxation.

Please note that I mentioned a stuffed animal, not an actual pet. Our pets, like our human companions, involve relationships—two-way streets that require care and cooperation.

Evaluate how your critters affect your sleep. Is your dog a faithful companion guarding your bedroom door or is he waking you several times in the night? Do your cats curl at your feet and warm your toes or are your toes a midnight toy?

I have a friend who house-sat a home with three small dogs. The owner requested that all three dogs sleep in the bed with her. Their up and down needs kept my friend's nights sleepless. No wonder the owners vacation frequently. It is the only time they get any rest.

Do not give in to your pets' whims at the expense of your sleep. You would recognize that a child who disrupts your sleep needs retraining and discipline. Your Chihuahua can handle it, too.

Avoid sleep medications. Their long list of dangerous side effects should be enough to deter anyone. My mother had a psychotic episode after taking a commonly prescribed sleeping pill. Instead, train yourself in sleep. Sleep clinics are also available.

If sleep remains elusive over a long period because of worry and difficulties, it is time to reevaluate the concerns that are stealing your sleep. Actively seek answers and help for the things in your life that need improvement. Work to make your life the best you can.

Sometimes, the solution is very difficult: "This marriage is over." "My child needs professional help." "I have to quit my job."

Yet, force-feeding a life that isn't working via busyness, denial, even drugs, is not the answer for a healthy life. Make the changes required to create a good life.

CHAPTER 11

Fatigue and Remembering to Forget

While healing the face, fatigue is common. Not only is stamina lost through the consequences of surgery, but the body is using extra energy to make repairs. Healing is emotionally draining, too. Stress, concern, and pain all add to fatigue.

For me, fatigue is a constant. That baseball not only rearranged my face; it also left me with a head injury. Like many folks with head injury, I now have trouble with fatigue.

Over the years, I have learned to optimize my energy. It is a bit like having a family budget. Things are going along fine, and then the old VW breathes its last. A new car is required, and so is a new monthly payment.

Your family budget is reduced. At first, it seems grueling and nearly impossible, but once you start cutting here and reducing there, you realize you can live quite well on your new budget. The trick is, you have to watch every dime.

I keep close track of my energy level, and I estimate and schedule expenditures accordingly. If I have paperwork to do, I know gardening needs to wait. If the garden is an unrecognizable weed patch, it's time to set my writing aside for a day or two so all my energy can go into physical labor.

When life's needs take me in all directions at once, I set priorities— and alarms. A hard lesson for me was learning to let things go. Prior to my accident, if I had a goal, I stuck with it. If that meant staying up until 2 a.m. to finish a project, so be it.

Gone are those days. Now I schedule increments of time for work, and when the increment expires, I stop working. An unfortunate result is that projects often take longer than I wish, and when they are completed, sometimes they are not up to the standard I had hoped, yet that is all my budget allows. I learned to live with it.

When I do stray and overextend my time, I've borrowed against tomorrow's energy. It's just like the dreaded credit card debt in the family budget. Not only is tomorrow's energy already used, but I owe interest on it as well. And the rates can be steep.

Let's say it's spring and I have planting to do in my garden. It is hard work, and I know four hours is the most time I should spend on it. Yet, while I'm working, I get a rhythm going; I feel strong, and tomorrow it might rain.

I keep pushing myself, and the next thing I know, seven hours of hard labor has gone by. That's only three hours more work, so it would seem a restful morning the following day would be suffice to recuperate.

Not so; there is interest to be paid. Pulling a stunt like that could cost days of needed rest, not hours. Mental exertion can be just as draining.

Sometimes I do overwork myself, despite the price to be paid. I plan for it in my schedule, much like one takes on major credit card debt to finance a new refrigerator. Yet, if I slip into energy debt on a whim, it is as foolish as running up a huge Visa bill, and having nothing to show for it.

Fortunately, I've learned ways to stay out of energy debt. First, I make a conscious effort to conserve energy. I try to make my environment quiet and peaceful by keeping stimuli to a minimum. Usually, I go without radio or music, opting for silence instead. Since I'm near-sighted, I can reduce visual stimuli simply by removing my glasses.

Next, I evaluate the cost of an activity. Staying late at the office, finishing the book, one more lap—all of those activities might be done without a second thought when one's energy is abundant, but not when energy is limited.

If I stay late at the office tonight, I will be dragging tomorrow. If I finish the book, I won't get enough sleep. Another lap will mean a light workout tomorrow because I won't have energy to do more.

I may decide all these activities are worth the energy expenditure. The important thing is I know the limitations of my energy, and I try to spend that energy wisely.

Learning to stop and come back later was another difficult lesson for me. I'm a housewife, and I like my kitchen clean at day's end. Yet an active day usually leaves me needing to relax after dinner, so my new routine is to clean the kitchen in the morning.

Another reason to stop and come back is that fatigue increases my chance of making errors. Mistakes, lack of focus, and irritability are all signs of being overtired. I've learned to shut off the computer. Tomorrow is another day.

When I have deadlines, I begin early and organize my time. Procrastination and fatigue do not mix.

Strong, toned muscles and a fit cardiovascular system allow energy maximization, thus maintaining fitness is an important expenditure. I am not a shining example of fitness, but I exercise almost every day. I choose my activity according to what my energy budget allows.

At a minimum, I take a brisk one-mile walk. At the maximum, I run in the Glenwood Hot Springs pool for 45 minutes plus another 45 minutes of isometrics and stretching.

Working out in water is easier on one's joints and energy usage and avoids straining muscles, yet my Glenwood workout is so intense that it takes energy planning, including a day of rest the following day.

My usual workout is dancing for 35 minutes plus stretching; my own combo of rock, hip-hop, and hula. I know how to dance as if no one is looking. I have not joined a gym because I am already disciplined about working out. Also, I tend to be competitive and social, both of which could strain my energy budget.

However, I have seen friends get terrific results from gym workouts. May I suggest, that if you have energy limitations, be aware of them while setting your gym program. Keeping up with the pace of a class, or steady increases in workout difficulty, might be an expense that is too high.

To conserve energy, I often try to relax my mind during exercise. In the past, I have faced severe fatigue while, at the same time, knowing I needed to exercise, so I developed a technique during walks I call "sleep walking."

I begin my walk and settle into a comfortable breathing rhythm. I then try to make my mind go blank, much like hypnosis. The longer I walk, the more I divorce my mind from my body.

My body is running efficiently, but my mind is shut off. I try to listen only to the sound of my breathing, making a conscious effort to tune out my environment. I can even close my eyes for short intervals. Obviously, a safe, flat walking surface is needed. I do not use treadmills or headphones.

When successfully executed, I complete my walk with muscles exercised and my mind, if not rested, at least not further taxed.

This idea of divorcing body and mind to conserve energy works for mental exertion as well. If I'm deep into a project at the computer, I try to make my body as comfortable as possible. I take deep breaths and focus on relaxing my muscles. I stand, stretch, and take quick walks to ward off tension.

I try to keep a good attitude toward my body by seeing it not as a nuisance that needs pampering, but as a worthy machine that sees me through the day.

Yet fatigue was not the only challenge that baseball presented me. It rattled my short-term memory as well. My memory, or lack thereof, can drain energy, because the more things I try to remember, the more energy I expend.

It's a bit like lugging the groceries into the house. With one bag in each hand and your purse over your shoulder, you're fine; but three more bags, a bottle of wine, and your backpack later, you're weighed down and ready to topple.

Luckily, I have discovered a tool that does much of the remembering for me—my smartphone.

If I have something to do in the afternoon, I set my smartphone alarm to tell me when to begin. That frees me from having to remember the event or even the time.

There are so many things my smartphone can remember in my stead. For example, I don't need to remember the date or the day of the week because my smartphone tells me. When I make plans for lunch with a friend, I don't need to remember conflicting appointments. Instead, I consult my calendar.

I discipline myself to put everything on my smartphone. As I make an appointment, I enter it on my phone. I put my grocery list there, too. Everything is automatically backed up on iCloud, so even if I lose or break my phone, the information is usually retrievable. I make hard-copy backups only for the most vital information or when I'm traveling.

There is much evidence to suggest that by turning off memory and concentrating on a single subject, mental ability can be increased. Many theorize this is one reason why individuals like Albert Einstein and Stephen Hawking are so smart.

Years ago I read about Alexander Graham Bell walking through the Boston University campus and coming upon some students. He joined them in a lively intellectual conversation and as he said goodbye, he asked, "Which way did I come from?"

The students pointed to the left. Bell said, "Good. Then I've had my lunch."

This man of great brilliance didn't remember if he had eaten. Instead, he was using his mind for more important matters. For those of us looking to save energy, Bell's example fits well; be miserly with your memory.

There are many ways to ease the need to remember. I always keep my car keys in a dish on the kitchen windowsill. I don't need to remember where I put my keys; they are always there.

In truth, it goes against my personality to be so rigid. I have an artistic personality that repels repetition, yet I have found my "one place" rule such a huge energy saver that I stick with it. My stuff has no special place and no temporary place; it has one place.

In opposition is clutter. Of all the drains on memory, clutter is the worst. Clutter demands that you keep track of everything at once, thus taking tremendous amounts of energy. And when you can't remember where things are, you exert physical energy that is often accompanied by energy-draining frustration in an effort to find it.

Disorganization creates the same pattern. Clutter also encourages overabundance, even hoarding, which also takes tremendous energy. Years ago my family and I visited Malta. One of the many things we loved about the place was grocery shopping. We bought our meat from the small butcher shop and produce from the vegetable stand. The selections were small and delicious.

When we returned home, I remember feeling overwhelmed by the supermarket. Good grief: How many kinds of toothpaste do we need?

Having so many choices isn't a privilege, it's a nuisance.

I can't help feeling the same about a friend's closet that overflows with clothes. There are so many choices that it takes my friend hours to decide what to wear. I have a relatively small closet with comparatively few outfits. In fact, when my closet gets too full, I force myself to get rid of some clothes rather than look for more space. For me, deciding what to wear is simple; it's either this, that, or the other. The more stuff I have, the more energy I waste dealing with it.

It's an easy conclusion for me: keep stuff to a minimum. My "one place" rule has become so much a part of me that I use it whenever I can, including when parking my car. I always try to park in front of the entry door of the business I'm visiting.

Parking being what it is, that isn't always possible, yet by applying my one place rule, it feels wrong if I park on the side. Following my rule makes remembering where I parked much easier.

Another tool I use for keeping track of locations is to take a picture with my smartphone. (I will add this tip: When traveling, especially in countries whose native language is not my own, I take pictures of bus stops, my hotel, and other important landmarks so I can show pictures when asking directions.)

I use all my senses as memory aids. When traveling I carry my own bags, and I try to have physical contact with each bag at all times, thus using my sense of touch to keep track of them.

For example, when walking, my purse is over my shoulder, my suitcase is at my side, and a carrier is in my hand. When I sit, the purse goes over my leg (more comfortable), the suitcase sits next to me so my left arm brushes it, and the carrier is at my right foot.

I don't have to think about my luggage because my sense of touch is keeping track of it. When I don't have contact with a piece, I feel something is missing, thus it is highly unlikely I will forget to grab my suitcase from storage.

Everything I carry has one place—not sometimes in my purse and sometimes in my suitcase. If I take something out I'm aware of the displacement, so when my laptop leaves my bag I'm not entirely relaxed until it's back in again. (Given how many laptops are left in airports each year, this, too, is a good travel tip.)

Again, I avoid clutter. I pack light.

Yet for all my work at outsourcing remembering to my smartphone, and the pride I take in learning how to cope with memory deficiency, I have to admit: Lack of memory can be embarrassing. I can't begin to count the times I've felt like a fool.

I've hurt friends' feelings, too, because sometimes my memory just doesn't work; and even though that person is important to me, an occurrence that has affected him or her never reached my memory banks, and I have no recollection of their dilemma. To them, it feels like I don't care.

Another embarrassment is that I have difficulty remembering faces, which also can be hurtful to others. Everyone is used to having their name forgotten, but not their face. Not remembering can make me feel like I appear uncaring and dumb. And if I don't allow myself adequate rest, things can get worse.

One more factor in my baseball mental rearrangement is that I don't have a built-in sense of time like most people do. Often, for me to recall whether something happened two weeks ago, two months ago, or last year takes using events that I do remember as tags and drawing a line back to the date I want to recall.

I don't have a good sense of minutes and hours passing either, which is another reason setting alarms is important. If I become severely fatigued, I drop into what I call "time warping," which makes time even less perceivable for me.

If I continue without allowing myself rest, I can start having blackouts. At first, these blackouts consist of short periods, usually a few minutes, of which I have little to no recollection. If I continue without rest (yes, I've actually done this), I can have long blackouts.

The first time this happened was when I was chairing our local toy drive. A woman called one day to confirm a host of information and scheduling she and I had set up a few days prior. I had no recollection of the conversation—or even of the woman. It frightened me and left me insecure about my mental ability.

Fortunately, the warning signs of fatigue blackouts are now obvious, and I've learned to heed the warnings. Only on a few occasions have I experienced blackouts.

Once, while severely fatigued, I came up against what Theresa Schneider, a friend with severe head injury, calls "the brick wall."

It happened during the holiday season. I parked on our main street, stepped out of my car, and a man in typical small town fashion said hello and asked how I liked my car.

"I love it," I said.

"What year is it?" he asked. Brick wall.

The car was scarcely a year old. I remembered that, but I had no recollection of what year it was—no recollection at all. It was a terrifying feeling. I tried hard to remember, but my mind was blocked by the brick wall. I tried narrowing down the number. I was sure the millennium had passed.

Maybe 2007—or did that sound too far in the future? Still the brick wall. No clue of the year was reaching me.

I don't remember what I said to the man. I only know that I got away from him quickly. I don't recall when the year returned to my memory; maybe ten minutes later—the year was 2014—but I do remember feeling terrified yet recalling the advice Theresa had given me years prior:

"When your memory hits a brick wall, don't try to climb over it. Work your way around it."

Theresa's advice made that terrifying moment more endurable. I knew that what was happening was the result of my head injury, and I knew it would pass. I did not feel alone. Luckily, the brick wall has not shown up again.

Let me conclude this chapter with a final note on fatigue: Hatred, anger, revenge, meanness—all of those take energy. Love, peace, forgiveness, and kindness take little. They can even help your energy grow.

CHAPTER 12

You Are What You Say

Fiction writers use descriptive tags to identify their characters. These tags are repeated frequently so that when readers hear "messy blonde hair," they know it's Joanne and "nervous cough" means Mike has arrived.

We, too, create tags. "I'm always on the go." "I'm a homebody." These repeated bits of information tell others who we are. Listen closely to what you say about yourself. "I'm a soccer mom," tells others you have children, and are devoted to them and their sport. "I'm fat" makes them check your waistline and tells them you are insecure about your appearance.

Be careful of the tags you plant. I have a friend who constantly calls herself "dumb." Though a bright woman, her repeated "dumb" tag makes her appear featherbrained and lacking in self-confidence.

Generally, I do not talk about my facial history. I don't want to be tagged "that poor woman who shattered her face." If I do tell my tale, it is after I have established myself as just plain Lois. As I mentioned in

Choosing Your Doctor, I met a gang of friends, the Trekkie family, before beginning my third reconstruction.

At the time, I felt deformed. Yet, this wonderful group of people seemed not to notice, or at least not be distracted by my appearance. I was simply Lois, a new friend.

I projected myself as normal, confident, even attractive and they accepted my projection. It was not until our relationship was established that I told my tale.

Whenever I share my facial history, I end with "Thank God, I'm still cute." This remark always solicits a smile and I hope I'm tagging myself with "a sense of humor" maybe even "cute" and not "that poor woman."

Be especially careful what you say to those closest to you. They do not need to hear a steady stream of negativity. Living with facial differences is difficult for you and your loved ones. They, too, have to adjust and accept. Hearing constant bemoaning about how bad you look makes it more difficult for everyone.

Discussions about struggles, hopes and fears can vent frustrations and build stronger relationships. Yet, even these discussions should be limited. When I was in the midst of surgeries, concern for my face dominated my life. Discussing the cares and concerns of everyday life became a grounding point for me and my husband, connecting us to the world and to each other.

What you say about yourself also affects how you feel. As I mentioned in Pain Relief, strolling down the memory lane of your pain can invoke unpleasant memories and even encourage pain's return. You can also encourage illness. Your mind tends to create the images you focus on, so if you focus on the flu you had last month, telling everyone the details, you are encouraging return of the symptoms, perhaps even the illness. There is a reason hypochondriacs are always sick.

Finally, be kind in your words to yourself. It is amazing the names I used to call myself: "stupid" "pathetic." I would never call someone else such names, so why myself? I am not alone in this. I think there is a perverse idea in our society that demoralizing ourselves keeps us from vanity.

I am cultivating a new attitude. I try to think of myself as my own best friend. If my best friend knocked over a glass of milk, I would not call her "idiot." I might teasingly say "smooth move," or even feel upset by the mess, but I would not belittle her. I am working to show the same verbal respect for myself.

You are what you say, so say nice things.

CHAPTER 13

Attitude—It May Not Be Everything, But It's Close

As a patient, the most important thing I brought to my surgeries and subsequent healing was a good attitude. Even my most stoic doctors commented on its positive effects. Maintaining a good attitude is not a simple task. Pain, fear and sadness are also part of the healing process. Yet, by focusing on the positive and working to be at peace and happy, my healing process was made a far better journey.

I rarely go without a smile. Most often, it comes naturally, but some days, like Joe Gideon in All That Jazz, I declare "It's show time" and force my smile into place. I had a great teacher.

My mother was a severe arthritic and at the end of her life, her body was twisted into a ball; yet, she generally maintained her good attitude. She loved Nat King Cole's "Smile" and Mom lived the lyrics. Though pain and difficulties plagued her, she put a smile in place and she worked to make it fit.

The attitude began with my grandmother, a stern Scottish woman of Victorian values. "Chin up. No complaining," was her motto. My mother took the next step; if your chin must be up and complaining is not allowed, you might as well smile.

Seeing beauty in the world helps build a positive attitude, too. Beauty is not just pretty flowers and majestic landscapes. It is the way light hits your coffee cup, the shape of a rock, the color of a pile of leaves. Beauty is with us in everyday objects; yet, we often do not notice.

If an artistic eye does not come naturally, a quick introduction to art can glean appreciation for shape, lighting, color and contrast; the foundations of visual beauty. To enhance my artist's eye, I photographed things around the house; simple things like salt and pepper shakers, my gardening hat on its hook. I had fun and the exercise awakened me to the allure of my surroundings.

There is beauty in sound, as well: bird songs, children's laughter, a whispered breeze. Every genre of music has unique and creative appeal. Silence, too, holds beauty. Touch can soothe or stimulate (e.g., the feel of wool, warm water poured over cold hands or a soft and warm kitten).

Despite all the challenges I faced, finding beauty in the world brought me peace and happiness.

Another ingredient to a positive attitude is to dip into the fountain of youth. Be assured, youth is more a state of being, than an age. One of my youngest (and dearest) friends just turned ninety. I know some tottery old codgers in their thirties.

Margaret, at ninety, is vivacious. She's optimistic. She tries new things, thinks new thoughts and listens to new ideas. Margaret likes to have fun. She's witty, rarely sarcastic and never belittling. She likes winning, but being king of the hill is not her main goal; she just wants to play. Margaret is interested—in me, in you, in life. "Been there, done that" is not a Margaret bumper sticker. She sees life as new every day.

The old codgers in their thirties are a different story. They are lethargic and pessimistic. They are set in their ways and convinced newness and change would be bad or not worth the effort. These old folks are dragged down by worries; immediate things like "I'll never get a raise" and long-term issues like spending their daughter's first birthday worrying about how to put her through college.

Old codgers love to worry and they are convinced nothing will go right. To them, everything is a chore.

My best days are when I see life as a playground. I have on my new red sneakers and the swing set is open—joy, hope, possibility. Of course, there are bullies around, and some nasty bruises to endure, but that's not where a kid's mind is when running onto the playground. She is thinking of the thrill of swinging high in the air and the amazing speed of new red sneakers.

That is youth. That is the fountain from which to dip.

Play—giggle yourself silly—play. Many adults scarcely remember how it's done; yet, play is a great tension relief valve. Children love recess and their teachers recognize the need of that joyful reset button. As adults, we still need that joy.

Laughing exercises our lungs. Play surges our endorphins. Look for fun and remember play is innocent wonder. Turn off criticism of yourself and others. Dismiss worries about what people might think. LOL, laugh out loud; make it a reality, not just a texting notation.

Another step in harnessing a good attitude: see positive, hear positive, speak positive. Many people fall into a habit of negativity. They watch the woes of the world on television; they listen to radio hosts ranting complaints then voice their own displeasure with practically every-thing. If negativity doesn't do the trick, there's always sarcasm.

Think about what you see and hear in a day; the television shows you watch, the articles you read. How much is negative? What about the things you say. Really listen to yourself. Do you sound upbeat or do you complain?

I have friends who, no matter what is said, make a negative remark. If I say it's a lovely autumn day, they respond, "But winter is just around the corner." They make these remarks to be witty or conversational, but that doesn't stop their negativity.

Gossip, too, darkens our attitude. I think of life as a pond and the things we do and say as pebbles thrown in, sending ripples on the water. When our words and actions are kind and positive, the ripples soothe but when we are negative and cruel, they send out anger and discourse.

If you know something bad about someone, keep it to yourself. Do not throw it out for others to scoff at or to create anger. To those who insist they must "tell it like it is," let me share as well. I have a bowel movement each day but I refrain from "telling it like it is" and giving details of its appearance. Perhaps we could all show the same courtesy. "A guard before my mouth and a watch before my tongue."

There are times when negativity gets overwhelming. I've dedicated the next chapter to dealing with sadness, but an angry mood can also detour a good attitude. When I'm in an angry snit, it is easy to blame everything and everyone. "Of course I'm angry—my face is a mess, I'm tired all the time, my best friend won't call me back, the cookies burned."

I can get a real laundry list going. Yet, just as pain has an epicenter, often, so too does an angry mood. I go through my laundry list as calmly and detached as possible. I try to see each irritant like a specimen under a microscope.

Most often, I find one thing that sends a particular shot of anger through me and frequently it is something small, the straw that breaks the camel's back. When I find the irritant, I do what I can to ease it, get rid of it, and when I have done all that is possible, I try to drop it. Dwelling on the irritant only stokes anger's fire.

Sometimes, anger needs to be vented, but words should be chosen carefully. Once said, words cannot be erased. Try to take anger out on something rather than someone, and when colliding with others, express anger with the problem not the person. Fight fair.

My priest advises to make your words needful, truthful and as kind as possible. Good advice. Stick to the present, too. Your significant other left the milk out today so let him know that pissed you off. He does not need to be reminded that he did the same thing eight weeks ago.

Work your way out of anger, and remember frustration and boredom are of the same family. Evaluate physical troubles that might be contributing to your anger. Just as your grandmother warned, constipation can sour your mood, so can PMS and lack of sleep.

Always do your best. If you do your best, whether you succeed or fail, you can walk away knowing you did what you could. Recently, I had to make a speech in front of a large audience. I hate public speaking and I am not good at it.

I spent a lot of time preparing my speech. I rehearsed for hours. I did my best. The speech did not go particularly well, but I can look back with full confidence that I did my best.

Many emotions have a positive effect on the healing process. Feeling twitterpated is the best emotion for healing I have found. Twitterpated is the feeling of excitement caused when that certain someone walks into the room. It is the butterflies in your stomach, the smile you cannot make go away. It's middle school all over again and your big crush just arrived at the dance.

Granted, you probably are not feeling your best, nor do you consider your appearance at best. Yet twitterpated, like all emotions, is a matter of mind, not circumstance. Adoration for a significant other can create a twitterpated feeling, and if those feelings have faded, try stirring them.

If not a significant other, look for someone you have a crush on or try remembering back to someone who gave you that twitterpated feeling. Relive it. Embrace it.

Aside from my husband, listening to wonderful Rat Pack songs performed by James Darren stir my twitterpated feelings. Once I have achieved that feeling, I turn it back on myself. I focus on seeing myself as lovable, desirable.

My appearance may be the ugly duckling, but I assure myself that inside me is the beautiful swan. I bask that swan in twitterpated feelings.

Some final thoughts for a positive attitude: First, happiness has almost nothing to do with circumstance. It took me years to realize this, and when I did, happiness became far more obtainable. In fact, most of the time, and despite the difficulties I've had, I am a happy person.

Many people live under the false assumption that circumstance is required to obtain happiness, as if being happy was the end reward. "I'll be happy when…" Yet, even when goals are met, often, happiness still alludes them. That is because happiness is a state of mind. It is not something that comes to you, but rather something you create via your thoughts and concentration.

If you want to be happy, focus on being happy. If given the choice of working yourself into a huff over a remark your sister made or letting it go and enjoying the sunset, choose the sunset.

Finally, live in the moment. In this moment, there is no past to look back on; no mistakes, mishaps or wrong turns to lament. In this moment, there is no future looming down with the fear of potential failures and disasters. At this moment, there is only now, and no matter where I find myself, I can smile because this moment is life and I am part of it.

CHAPTER 14

Embracing Sadness

As you recall, I am a uniform-wearing, never-miss-a-Vegas-con," Trek-kie. Only by attending a Star Trek convention can one conceive of how crazy fun they are; parties every night with folks from all over the world, all walks of life, in a festive atmosphere that reflects Star Trek's enthusiasm for coexistence.

A few years ago, my convention was disrupted by sadness. I had lost my sister a few months earlier, and though not an unexpected passing, nonetheless, it was difficult. I was also in flux about my facial surgeries. It was mid-convention, the two biggest parties of the year that night, and at 4 pm I informed my gang I needed space.

I locked myself in my room. I curled up on the bed with my stuffed animal, Fudd, and I cried. I ordered in dinner and breakfast and I did not emerge until the next afternoon.

Sadness had paid a visit and I knew to drop everything, even the highlight of my year, and tune in.

Aside from fun, the Star Trek convention is a milestone, a way I review my year. I always arrive at conventions like a kid, playing tag, rushing to base and shouting, "Safe!"

That convention, I staggered in. It had been a grueling year. I'd had my eye eviscerated. I was still adjusting to life with my prosthesis. In addition, I'd had another facial surgery, which had yet to please me. Most compelling was my grief from losing my sister.

Hell of a year. I was pent up and upset. I was deeply saddened.

When reconstructing the face, or going through whatever difficulties life casts, waves of sadness will hit. They are part of the healing process.

These waves remind me of when I went body surfing as a teenager. I was warned that if a wave dragged me down, not to fight it, but to ride it out. I was doing well and feeling cocky when out of nowhere, a huge wave slammed me down to what felt like Davy Jones' locker.

Panic surged in me, and I curled into a ball. The power of the water was unbelievable—frightening, overwhelming—then I was thrown onto the shore. By the time I sat up, the wave had slipped back and I was on bare ground.

My convention experience felt like that. Sadness hit me fast and hard, yet, I knew to curl up and ride it out. When I emerged from my room the next day, I was ready to rejoin the fun. My friends expressed concern, but I could honestly tell them my sadness and my need to be alone were a part of the healing process.

All was well.

It is my experience that when sadness comes pounding at your door, you should embrace it. If you feel yourself gasping for air, curl tighter. Live only that moment and its sadness—no future, no past. If you are bewildered by a new appearance, grab it, hold on to it; just the two of you locked in space without time.

No bemoaning the good old days of a "normal" face, no grieving a future with a face you dislike. Allow only the present, the now, that face and you, until sadness recedes. It will recede, if you give it the attention it needs.

Do not try to push unresolved sadness away. You will waste your energy. Do not try outrunning it with busyness. It will catch up to you. Postponing sadness until a more convenient time is equally unadvisable. When sadness hits, let it take its course.

Brace yourself and let it work through you. When it subsides, swim for shore. It's better to take the waves of sadness as they come, than let them build into a tidal wave.

I firmly believe that by embracing sadness as it appeared, I warded off depression, a difficulty that once plagued me. Years ago, I fought with depression and it manifested into panic disorder. There were times I could hardly leave my house.

My husband and I sometimes discuss how I got over my depression and we both agree—the baseball did it. Perhaps not entirely, but that ball played a major role.

Along with the damage it did to my face, I also suffered head injury. I now have trouble with fatigue and I have little sense of time, both long and short term. I also have memory loss. There is a significant downside to memory difficulties, but it has one great asset:

I forget to worry.

My mother was a worrier, so I grew up believing being worried equated to caring. I took that worry and blew it out of proportion—spending time either going back over my humiliating mistakes or forward to terrifying possibilities. It made me depressed and resulted in panic disorder.

After that baseball short- circuited my memory, I had to make an effort to remember to contemplate the negativity of past and future. I eventually found it dysfunctional and stopped fretting. I am now one of the happiest, least depressed people I know, including my times of sadness.

Living the moment helps defeat depression, too. Depression does not live well in the moment—he likes things to chew on—bad memories, fears. Give him just the moment and he loses strength.

Another important anti-depressant is to love thy neighbor. Life is good when we follow this advice. Respect for others breeds peace. Kindness harbors love.

When you're feeling down, can't get up, at the end of your rope; send a get- well card to a sick friend, help a stranger find directions, volunteer at a charity rummage sale.

Depression demands self-centered attention. Pull away from yourself by thinking of, and doing for, others. Love thy neighbor is the best antidepressant on the market.

Sadness and depression are a part of life. They are among the experiences that make life complete. They are the dishes at the banquet we do not want to try, the ones that make us pucker. Yet, afterward, when the banquet is complete and we are sipping brandy, we realize the meal was better—fuller, richer—because of them.

CHAPTER 15

Helpers in Healing

When healing, the people in our lives are more than loved ones, confidants and companions. They are also our helpers in healing. We can optimize their help by deducing what we need from them and guiding them toward that goal.

After my accident, I was horribly rattled. I had not been home from the hospital long when my husband and son had to go out of town for a few days.

I was not ready to be alone. I thought of the people I knew whom I could spend time with to lift my spirits. I called a woman I knew more casually than well ,and who was forty years my senior. When I asked Margaret if I could spend the day with her, I could tell she was surprised, perhaps leery, but she agreed. It was the beginning of a beautiful friendship.

I chose Margaret for several reasons. First was availability. Margaret was retired and most of my friends were working moms. Yet, it was more than that. I wanted to be with someone who was not intimately involved in my calamity. I craved the company of someone outside of my crashed world. In addition, Margaret has a wonderful personality. I wrote about her in my chapter on attitude. She is vivacious, interested, and therefore, interesting. Margaret is fully alive.

I needed someone fully alive to keep me in the moment. My world was in turmoil; I was pulverized and weak. Twice, an artery in my nose broke loose, and both times, I feared I would bleed to death. I had yet to learn if my eye could be saved. Amid all of this was my remorse for dragging my ten-year-old son and husband through the chaos.

The last thing I needed to think about was where I had been or where I was going. I wanted to discuss art and music. I wanted to laugh at some crazy story from Margaret's life. I needed the enjoyment of the moment.

I needed Margaret.

When possible, choose your company and guide the conversations. Often, people want to show their concern by sympathy. Keep these conversations brief because sympathy is one of the worst things you can get.

While expressing fears and worries can vent some nasty feelings, it can also lock you into a "woe is me" trap that gets you nowhere. After a few kind words of sympathy, try changing the conversation. Ask about their life; the fun, everyday side of their life. Use your time with others to get away from your dilemma.

This is also an ideal time to discuss ideas and quandaries you have reached via contemplation. Does life happen in random chaos or is there purpose to each step? What is the meaning of life?

You may be surprised who is interested in such conversations and their views may be unexpected as well. One precaution: many people during healing reach new heights in their religion and spirituality. These experiences can be uplifting, even euphoric, and it is natural to want others to have that same feeling. However, while sharing your spirituality and religion may make interesting conversation, rarely do others want a sermon. Be conversational not didactic.

Your situation is not just difficult for you, but for your loved ones as well. Be particularly mindful of those closest to you, especially children. Try for balance; be appreciative of their shoulder to cry on, yet, not overburdening. Show strength, but don't try to hide your difficulties. Often, people don't know what to say and their unsureness can make them hesitant to be around you. In the beginning, they may also find your appearance too difficult to accept and avoid you. Be understanding of their difficulty, and again, when you are with loved ones, guide the conversation. In general, try keeping to the lighter side of life. During the healing process, you may be isolated from an active life. Try living vicariously through your interest in other people's lives; their daily challenges, hobbies and children.

One of my dearest friends and I regularly share whimsies. It is a fun means of distracting us from day-to-day life. We are on the watch for things that make us chuckle and shake our heads, like the man with a backward cap who cups his hand over his eyes to block the sun.

Share the humor of everyday life. Reach into yourself for strength, too, and try showing your loved ones that though your road is difficult, it is doable. This will ease their discomfort and doing so builds your inner strength.

At times, I was bewildered by what I felt was a lack of sympathy and understanding, particularly during my third reconstruction. My husband said it was my own fault. "You're always upbeat and act like you're doing fine. How are people supposed to know you need sympathy?"

I had to admit, he was right.

As I said in my chapter on attitude, I project myself as strong, able to cope and happy. I don't always feel that way, but by acting so, I gain strength. While I may have wished for more concern, if given the choice, I would rather be perceived as a person who doesn't need sympathy than someone who does.

Yet, there were many times I went to my friends for comfort. I was blunt about my fears and sorrow. Sometimes, I would curl into a friend's embrace and say, "I need you to tell me everything is going to be all right."

I learned quickly with whom I could share my feelings. In addition, just as each person is unique, so too, were their responses. I learned whom to seek out when I needed to be washed in compassion or distracted, and who to see when I needed my backside kicked.

A few times the response I received was so unlooked for, I felt crushed. Prior to beginning my third reconstruction, I had reunited with several cousins. I was looking forward to their support in beginning my third reconstruction.

That is not what happened.

I received a unanimous condemnation of my pending reconstruction as frivolous and vain. I was angry about what I perceived as their trivialization of my deformity and our relationship suffered. Yet, even this had a positive note. Through my anger and frustration with them, I looked deeper into myself and strengthened my resolve.

Be prepared; people will say the darnedest things. "At our age, it doesn't matter what we look like," one man told me. "Your eye used to really bother me, but I've gotten used to it," a woman remarked.

Worst were the "if it were me, I wouldn't care how I looked." —I heard this from many people and I never believed a single one of them.

A dear friend said, "I think you're addicted to surgery."

Ouch.

The truth is, during my final reconstruction, I kept moving forward, one surgery after another, because I knew from my accident that once I stopped and let myself smell the fresh air above the trenches, I wouldn't go back.

Addicted to surgery? I loathed it. No one will ever understand how much courage it took for me to face the knife again and again.

For good or bad, people play an important role in our healing process. They are our mirrors, reflecting their perceptions of us. Upbeat friends and family rally us with positive reflections. They stir hope, happiness and bring sunshine to dark days. They see our beauty. Other friends can bring us down with pessimism and their bemoaning of how "unfair" it all is, or worse, trivializing the situation.

From a healing standpoint, spending time with the upbeat and not with the downcast is best, but rarely is this possible. Nor would we want it to be. Gloomy though they may be, the downcast are also friends and family. We love them. We want to be with them.

Like all things in life, balance is the best solution. The hard truth is, during the healing process, it is best to limit your exposure to gloomy people. This is often not easy, and can be hurtful to those around us.

During my initial cancer surgeries, my husband's parents, who were in their nineties and needing care, were a constant concern and there was the worry that soon they would need to go into a nursing home. Yet, despite their needs and our worries, I limited my time with them and I did not allow myself to think about them very much.

This may sound hard, but I knew getting myself well was top priority. It's as the airline attendant says, "Get your own oxygen mask on before helping others."

A positive attitude was the most important tool I had in my healing process. It was my lifeline. If I allowed attitudes and circumstances of others to bring me down, I was doing myself a disservice. I evaluated the situation, figured out how far I could limit time with my in-laws and I stuck to my plan.

Limit time with the perpetually pessimistic, too. You know the type; if it hasn't gone wrong yet, it will. Others are caught in dire circumstances that make them downcast and perhaps saddest are those who are clinically depressed. These are all people we love, people who it is our duty to help as family, friends, or if nothing else, fellow human beings, but the hard truth is, limiting your exposure to these people is best while healing.

You may also realize, as I did, that you have unhealthy relationships that need to be greatly limited or ended. After thirteen years of helping a very demanding elderly woman, for my own physical and mental health, one day I said, "No more."

Sometimes it is the only way. Honestly evaluate the situation. Do not let others, or yourself, fill you with guilt. When healing, you need to focus on yourself. If others cannot understand this, as the old psychology adage goes, they own the problem.

CHAPTER 16

Working with a Team of Doctors

Reconstructing the face can require the expertise of several doctors, with your lead doctor coordinating their efforts. As stated in an earlier chapter, you need a lead doctor with whom you have confidence. I think of him as head coach, knowing what to do and which players to use to get the job done.

As patients, we rely on our doctor to see us to our goal. Yet, this does not mean we stay on the sidelines. We know ourselves and our bodies better than anyone does, and that information, along with what we hope to achieve, is essential knowledge for a good game plan.

If your lead doctor seems hesitant or unwilling to bring in someone with more expertise, that's a red flag. If the needed procedure is simple or within his field, he probably has a valid point, but if extensive or intricate reconstruction outside his field is required, experts are advised.

Be assertive about getting the right person for the job. Make sure your lead doctor's primary concern is making you look your best, not his opportunity to do the surgery.

Keep your doctors apprised of each other's work, especially your lead doctor. Do so quickly, precisely and leave appropriate information for their charts. A picture is worth a thousand words.

My neck was fused between surgeries with my guru doctor in Tucson. Instead of telling him about that surgery, I showed him a picture of the plate in my neck. It was a fast, easy way to give him the information he needed.

Rarely is your lead doctor your primary doctor; thus, your lead doctor is probably not watching your general health, nor is it his responsibility. Therefore, it is important to stay connected with your primary doctor. Keep her informed. Make sure she receives reports on all of the procedures you have done. Have periodic checkups with your primary doctor to ensure your general health is good and whenever possible, have pre-surgery tests, such as EKGs and blood work, performed via your primary doctor.

When seeing your primary doctor, briefly discuss work done to date and other procedures you have planned. Just as important, be your own doctor. Monitor your health and keep records of all your tests and reports.

When meeting with your doctors, project yourself as a competent member of the team. Be informed. Try to look your best. Be friendly and optimistic, and show enthusiasm for the work ahead. If you have fears and misgivings, by all means discuss them, but try to do so with an attitude of overcoming obstacles, not foreboding doom.

If a doctor fails to see the goal you want to reach, consider replacing him. After my accident and first reconstruction, I visited an ophthalmologist I had seen prior to my accident. At that time, I had my natural eye, and though it had been greatly traumatized, it was stable and doing well. The ophthalmologist suggested I start wearing a patch over my eye.

I was flabbergasted. So much work and energy had gone into saving my eye that to me it was a prized jewel, not something to hide. In addition, though the sight in my eye was then very limited and caused double vision, it was still sight, something to treasure, not block.

Finally, did he think my appearance was so unpleasant that I'd look better as a pirate? I was outraged. Upon returning home, I wrote him a letter explaining why he was being fired. I never saw him again.

CHAPTER 17

Stop or Go? Debating More Surgery

The truth is, you will probably not be thoroughly, or perhaps even mostly, pleased with your face if you experience extensive damage. Even guru doctors are limited. Therefore, it is important to set realistic goals for your appearance. To look "normal," to fit in without drawing attention, is a good starting place. Looking just as we did prior to surgery is rarely possible. Often, we can come close, making that another viable goal, but some changes are likely.

I miss my original nose.

It's funny, because as a teenager, I didn't like my nose. It was sharp with a bump at mid-bridge. I considered it too severe. My nose now is broader and without the chiseled appearance. It took a lot of expertise and numerous surgeries to get my nose to look as good as it does today and I am grateful. Yet, to me, it looks very different than it once did.

I miss my old nose.

How far you are willing to go to reach the appearance you want is a decision that takes a lot of thought. Seeking the opinions of both professionals and loved ones is a good idea. Yet, ultimately the decision should be yours.

As you go through surgeries and watch your face heal, you will get a sense of what can be done. Spend time at the mirror considering what procedures could improve your looks.

As I said, my final surgery was a face-lift and touch up of several areas. It was a surgical idea I came up with, not my doctors. My face is not very symmetrical and prior to that final surgery, one side of my face looked older than the other, accentuating the problem.

The face-lift brought better symmetry. One surgery after another, I kept moving forward to reach the goal I envisioned for myself.

I felt different after my accident. Then I was mom to a young son and anxious to get back to life. Though I was concerned with my appearance, it was not my top priority.

After my orbital blowout repair, my doctors suggested another surgery to fill the depression in my cheek. I quickly declined. I didn't want any more time spent in surgery. I was willing to live with my appearance, though more improvements could have been made.

There is much to consider when pondering further surgery. Time and money must be taken into account, risks as well. Surgeries are stressful not just to ourselves but also to our loved ones, so their feelings must be considered also. Guts and determination are required to go through multiple surgeries. Not everyone can endure it.

I know a man who went through numerous, painful surgeries trying to repair his hand. He is a wonderful man, but not strong of character. The surgeries drained him, oppressed him. He couldn't withstand the fight. In the end, his surgical odyssey was not successful and he became addicted to painkillers.

When considering multiple surgeries, be honest with yourself about your ability to endure pain, a brutalized appearance, down time and the jarring effects of adjusting to a new face. You must be willing to confront failure and disappointment, too. If you have a tendency toward addiction, this needs to be considered.

As you search and ponder, there will undoubtedly always be one more nip or tuck that would improve your looks; yet, at some point, you need to say "enough." If you are seeking new doctors because your current doctors advise against a procedure you want, you might be going too far. If loved ones who understood and previously supported your surgical goals are now opposed to more work, you may need to follow their advice.

Improving the face via surgery can become obsessive. Beware.

One logical solution might be to wait. Give yourself a few years of rest before deciding if further surgery is advisable. Personally, this is not something I would be able to do. For me, it was a matter of setting a goal and marching toward it.

I hated facing every surgery, but I kept moving forward. I was not stopping until my goal was reached. When that last surgery was performed, I was singing the *Alleluia!* chorus. I was done; there was no going back. Postponing the decision about future surgery would have hung over my head and disrupted my life.

We are unique. We each have individualized strengths and weaknesses. This, as well as our health, finances, time, impact on loved ones and our lifestyle need to be deliberated before doing more surgery.

While I said you might not be pleased with your facial appearance, you still should work to accept your face with as much love and appreciation as you can muster, no matter what stage you are in or how deformed you might feel. You and your face have withstood an ordeal.

Take pride in that.

LIVING WITH THE NEW YOU

CHAPTER 18

Facing Change

Adjusting to change after life-rattling events can be a bit like going through a body transformation. Once the initial shock subsides, we realize a lot of our jeans no longer fit. It is time to sort through the closet.

Some interests and activities may not be feasible at the moment. A brutalized appearance can be uncomfortable in public, leading us to spend more time at home. Pain and low energy can knock us out of other activities, but we can feel confident they will fit our lifestyle again soon. Some interests may no longer be possible.

After my accident, and the loss of vision in my left eye, I quit playing racquetball. I loved the sport, but a few nasty collisions with my partner convinced me I wasn't safe to play against.

There may be relationships and activities that no longer appeal to you. Perhaps they haven't for some time, or even never did. It is easy to get trapped into habits that do not bring us pleasure. Forced change is an opportunity for reevaluation. Avoid frustration by first acknowledging some change after a calamity is inevitable, and second, by taking it slow and figuring out what now fits in your life.

Whom you spend time with may change as well. Just because a person is a good friend, doesn't mean they will become a good helper in your healing process. If you sense a friend is struggling with your new needs, try involving them less. You might be disheartened, feeling like they don't care about you. Yet, for whatever reason, they may be unable to fulfill your needs.

Think about the relationship you had with this person prior to your calamity. If it was fun and stimulating, yet, lacked depth, it may be an unrealistic expectation to think this person will automatically join you in a serious and more demanding friendship.

Perhaps there is someone you helped, not asking anything in return, until now. Don't assume that your turn has arrived. If the relationship has always been one way, the other person may not be willing, or able, to return the kindness.

You can save yourself a lot of confusion and anguish by realizing friendships don't necessarily mold to your needs. Banging your head against a wall, trying to get help via a relationship that didn't include help before, can be hurtful and an upsetting waste of time.

If friends start pulling away from you, let them go. They may need to take a break to adjust to your new needs or they may not return. The decision is theirs. Yet, take heart. Almost inevitably, you will also find relationships that were casual or even passing, that suddenly become deeper, richer friendships.

There are people who are drawn to caring about and helping others. They enjoy the depths of life. Be open to these people. Don't be surprised by shifts in your friendships. Instead, try to be accepting of relationship changes.

It's a funny thing, change. Logically, we know the only constant in life is change. Yet, it can feel uncomfortable, even frightening, especially when it is thrust upon us. My experiences have taught me to take it slowly.

I have two personality traits that help me face forced change. First, I can be adventurous. Part of me fears change as many folks do. Yet, another part gets an inkling of excitement. I foster that excitement and encourage myself to feel "the game is afoot."

I see change as pushing my canoe out into an unfamiliar river (or as in the case with my accident and cancer, being launched without warning.) Part of me wants to dash back to shore. Yet, I make myself paddle out to deep water, for it is there that life flows. In the depths, I admit things have changed and I let it sweep me along.

Things start to happen. Life. It's the same reason I enjoy traveling, especially when I go alone. I meet new people, see new things, and because I am a sojourner in deep water, everything seems to take on a deeper meaning. I can feel it in those around me, for there are other sojourners out there. It is the lady I chatted with in the grocery store line, the teenager who delighted me with his exuberance, the rose that was the most radiant pink I had ever seen.

Change, especially unprepared for, wakes you up. If you fight change, fearfully clinging to the shore, you will miss the connection. You cannot fully experience an adventure you resist entering. When life hands you change, even if it is grueling and unpleasant, it's time for serendipity, or as it is called in Yiddish, *berrsheara*.

Things just happen if you relax and let the waters take you in a new direction. Not all of your experiences will be good, but that, too, is life.

Even the most reluctant armchair tourist has some sense of adventure. Foster your adventurous side when dealing with change.

Another trait that sees me through unexpected change: I am Vulcan.

Mr. Spock would be hard-pressed to outdo my cold, analytical side when it appears. In part, I think it is protection. I withdraw my emotions and look coldly, logically at what is happening. It enables me to make better, quicker decisions. It creates a buffer.

As I wrote in my chapter on embracing sadness, there is time when emotional hardship must be dealt with, but my cold, analytical side serves me well during immediate problems and as a break from my emotions. Yet, there is more to my Vulcan side than a protective shield. Even my most grueling physical difficulties I found "fascinating."

When I learned a piece of coral would be placed in my eye socket to help build an eye, I was intrigued. I was captivated by the pieces of my ears that were used to reconstruct my face. I am a living, breathing science experiment.

We all are. Find fascination in the changes you confront.

As you go through your healing process, you will hear a lot about recovery; yet, it is a word I have not used until now. To me, I did not recover from my accident, nor did I recover from my cancer.

I survived, I suffered, I endured, I learned, I grew and I became the woman I am today.

I do not consider that recovery. I see recovery as an attempt to go backward and regain a life that existed before earth-rattling events took place.

For me, recovery was impossible and unwanted. When I tried to go back and live as if no change had taken place, I felt uncomfortable, exhausted, and at times, like the proverbial square peg rammed into a round hole.

Like it or not, calamity changed my life. In a split second, that baseball brought change. I didn't look the same. My vision had changed so I saw the world differently. More profoundly, I had changed inside, not only because of my face but also due to subsequent head injury.

There were little things—prior to my accident, I loved Jazz, afterward I wanted to listen almost exclusively to concert music. Luckily, I again enjoy Jazz, but it took years.

There were big things—fatigue became a debilitating problem and my memory can be poor and unpredictable. I found myself in a new reality. I continue to adjust to the changes.

I wrote a short story long ago that was summarized by the main character: "If you begin life as one person, and end it as the same person; have you really lived?"

Life is change. It may be brought about through calamity that turns your world upside down. It may be via the slow tick of time. Yet, whatever the route, life is lived best when we embrace the riches, both simple and difficult, that change brings.

CHAPTER 19

Making the Most of Your Appearance

Your surgeries are over and your face has settled. The long struggle is over, but don't think the ability to improve your facial appearance has ended as well—far from it.

I see the time after surgical completion like a mother coming home from the hospital with a new baby. Finally, all the wonderfully helpful, poking, probing people are gone and you can settle in, just the two of you. I hope you've been working with your face all along. Now is the time to fine tune.

The first place to look for enhancement is at the muscles in your face and how they can be used to best maximize your appearance.

I have a slight paralysis on my upper left lip, which makes my smile crooked. As I stated in my chapter on attitude, I consider a smile an invaluable asset, so making my smile as pleasant as possible is important to me. I learned to use the muscles next to my nose to pull up my lip, thus, making my smile even. These are the same muscles used to snarl. It took a long time to zero in and train them. In fact, I don't have the same mobility with the muscles on my right side.

Learning to use these muscles independently took practice and my practice paid off. The left side of my mouth now has a fine tuned, automatic reaction. In fact, not flexing those muscles to smile now takes concentration.

Currently, I am working with the muscles around my left eye. My prosthetic eye does not have the same movement as the right and there are times my eyes appear out of synch. For example, when I look down, there is little to no change to my left eye, giving the appearance of one eye looking down and the other looking forward. To ease this appearance, I am trying to train myself to partially close my left eyelid when looking downward.

I hope with practice, it will become habit, just like my smile.

While we are on the subject of muscle use, examine your expressions, especially the involuntary ones, and see if there is room for improvement. Cringing the face, making the muscles highly flexed, can create an anxious expression and promote lines. A dropped jaw can cause a puzzled, or even foolish, look.

A lady at the optic shop I go to has the habit of squinting and curling her upper lip when she gazes at something close up. It is a most unpleasant expression, and it's obvious she has had this habit for a long time because she has developed lines from the gesture. It seems unfortunate to me, because she is a congenial woman and otherwise quite attractive.

Many external things can enhance your appearance, with glasses heading the list. In fact, even if you do not need glasses, you might consider wearing them. Keep in mind your needs in using glasses to enhance your appearance may be different from the norm. Usually, glasses are used to accentuate the eyes. That is exactly what I do not want.

My glasses have framing only at the top, not all around, which creates less accent for my eyes. In addition, the dark upper line of the glasses is near my eyes. This also gives less accent to my eyes and the strong line implies symmetry. Prior to my evisceration, I wore my glasses slightly tinted. This provided help for my fully dilated eye and made my eyes less noticeable.

Your hair frames your face so make sure it's styled to your advantage. Often, hair is styled to make a solid frame. I want a loose frame, so as a dear stylist said long ago, "We'll make it messy."

I try not to have any definite lines and just a wisp of bangs, or none at all. Due to nerve damage on my forehead, bangs can feel an itchy annoyance. I try to lift and push my hair back, keeping it feathery, and "messy."

I was born a blonde and have always been a blonde, but for a few years, I decided to try red. It was fun; yet, I had to be careful to not go too dark. My solution was to use blonde highlights.

When considering color, think lighter rather than darker, as lighter can seem softer and create less contrast, (unless you are very dark skinned). A natural looking color is advisable as it helps create a balanced appearance, rather than calling attention to anything, including your hair.

I've seen some beautiful silver grays and my mother-in-law had lovely snowy, white hair. Yet for many folks with gray hair, I think it looks dull and adds years. As an elderly, yet very attractive, female friend once told me, "If you want to stay young, never let your hair go gray."

I tend to agree with her, though I will note, my perpetually youthful friend, Margaret, has beautiful white/gray hair. Whatever you decide for your hair, think it through. If you are spending so much time and anguish rebuilding your face, give it a good frame with the right hairstyle.

Makeup is another great asset and I know men as well as women who use it to their advantage. Before my third reconstruction, my face was heavily scarred, so I used a liquid makeup so opaque, it was almost like theater paint.

I worked to make it as natural looking as possible, but in daylight, it was obvious I was wearing makeup. It was an appearance price I was willing to pay.

Which leads to an important discussion: What is the balance between working with your appearance and overworking it? Reactions to you are a good clue.

If you are wearing heavy makeup and people keep giving you second glances, you are probably overdoing. Some friends, the ones we both love and want to strangle, will quickly voice disapproval if we overdo. Yet, there is a greater concern aside from overdoing something.

You do not want to become so accustomed to a well-worked appearance that you become uncomfortable, even ashamed, of your natural look.

Years ago, before the evisceration of my left eye, I wore a contact over my eye. The contact gave me a bit more sight, but mostly, it improved my eye's appearance. As I mentioned, after my accident, my pupil was oddly shaped and fully dilated. Since I have light blue eyes, the deformity of my pupil was very noticeable.

The contact was quite a masterpiece; custom painted just for me; yet, it was delicate, too. It would fade over a fairly short period, making my eyes appear different hues. In addition, the contacts could tear easily.

They were high maintenance and expensive.

I felt like I looked much better with my contact, which boosted my confidence. Before wearing my contact, there were those uncomfortable initial introductions when a new acquaintance would notice (and try not to notice) my eye.

The discomfort would pass, and if I continued seeing the person, they often forgot about my eye. Yet, the odd appearance of my eye was always a distraction—except, when I wore my contact. Even when the contact faded and appeared a bit different color, it still improved the look of my eye.

Sometimes, I had to go without the contact. My eye would become irritated and need a break from it. I hated those days and I hated the double takes I got from people who were used to seeing me with a normal eye, and now a deformed eye.

The problem peaked during my son's high school graduation. There were so many activities, and though my son was the star, all we moms were under the spotlight, too. In the midst of the many festivities, my contact ripped. I didn't have a spare.

Thrust into the world without my contact, I felt like I was under the limelight, my deformed eye center stage. I felt humiliated and ashamed. Then I got angry. I grabbed my bootstraps and took the next step.

My son's graduation was one of the most exciting, crazy, beautiful times in his life; at least in the years I got to be by his side. I was not going to let the appearance of my eye disrupt it. If wearing a contact had taught me to be ashamed of my eye, it was wrong for me, and it needed to go.

I never wore a contact again. Don't let your enhanced appearance become so important that you feel uncomfortable, or even ashamed, of your natural self.

Another important aspect to boost your appearance is clothing. Our best outfit puts a spring in our step. That shirt that makes us feel like the Pillsbury Dough Boy can leave us self-conscious. Choose clothing that makes you feel confident. Be neat in your appearance, too. Few things encourage and project confidence better than a well-kept appearance.

Comfort is important. If your feet are miserable, you will be miserable, and your expression will show it. Do not be a victim of fashion either. Just because micro-short, spandex skirts are the rave, doesn't mean they are right for you.

If a fashion doesn't work for you, no matter how popular, don't wear it. Besides, wearing clothing a bit different from the masses can make you stand out. If you've chosen an outfit that works for you and you feel confident about, you will enjoy the attention.

The colors we wear can effect not just our appearance, but also our mood. I am sensitive to color and I enjoy wearing bright pastels. They cheer me, though, admittedly, they aren't always my best color choice. I am a busty woman and bright, light color tends to accentuate that. Yet I love the gladdened feeling I get, so I wear bright pastels anyway.

My son and many of his generation are wearers of black. While most of my pants and skirts are black, I rarely go without other color except for evening attire. Wearing black can make me lethargic and solemn. For others, I think black gives them confidence and boosts their ego.

We are all unique. When choosing clothing, think not just about how you look, but how your clothing makes you feel, too.

CHAPTER 20

It's All About Projection

As a Trekkie, my favorite place in the galaxy was Star Trek: The Experience at the Las Vegas Hilton. One step transported you from the thrill of Las Vegas to the intrigue of Star Trek's space station, Deep Space 9. There were rides that pitted you against Klingons and Borg, a restaurant with powerful, steaming drinks, and of course, merchandise.

As stated earlier, I got to know a lot of people via The Experience, and I treasure their friendships. I also treasure the lesson I learned from the actors at The Experience—the importance of projection.

Acting at The Experience was not your average gig. The actors did not learn their lines and take center stage. Instead, they researched their characters, endured the long process of makeup and wardrobe, then stepped into the crowd. Like Forrest Gump and his chocolates, they didn't know what they would get.

I loved being in the gift shop when an actor entered. Shoppers, deep in buying mode, were suddenly faced with a Klingon or conniving Ferengi. They might receive shopping advice from a blue Andorean or attempt small talk with a Vulcan. I saw some crazy reactions to the actors, but I never saw the actors break character. Consistently, I watched people accept that, yes, this was an alien from the world of Star Trek.

Yet, why did people accept them as aliens, I wondered. Admittedly, they were all good actors and their costuming was superb, yet, what sealed the deal? As I watched, I realized their secret—projection. They projected themselves as their character and those around them believed their projection. Through all the facial changes I endured, nothing helped more than this valuable lesson— how you project yourself is how people will see you.

As early as the completion of my third cancer surgery, I would throw my shoulders back, put a smile on my face and project myself as perfectly normal, even attractive. To my continued amazement, people usually accepted my projection. Most baffling was my annual visit to the Star Trek convention.

I was facing people I saw just once a year. Surely, they would notice the grueling changes; yet, most seemed unaware. Discussing this with friends at home, we decided the Trekkies were just being polite; yet I learned later, this wasn't true.

As my Trekkie friendships deepened, I began telling them about my facial reconstructions. Most of them seemed genuinely surprised to learn about it, and further, they generally had not noticed the extent of my deformities. At the 2014 Star Trek convention, I spoke during a panel about The Experience. I told the audience about my face and how invaluable I found the lesson in projection the actors taught me.

Afterward, a man who became my friend the year prior to my cancer diagnosis and whom I had spent time with every convention since, said to me, "I never noticed anything different about your face."

Admittedly, steeling myself to emanate confidence was easier said than done. To help, I often used a trick my friend, Francine, calls "the Mirror."

The Mirror is not the image reflected back to you from the wall. Rather, the mirror is a mental image that reflects the positive view of yourself you would like to see. It says, "Yes, you've gained weight, but you still look great" as opposed to the wall's, "When did that happen? You look terrible!"

The wall puts my scars under a spotlight, but the mirror says they barely show. The mirror generally finds my appearance more energetic, too. Which is telling the truth? It doesn't matter. What does matter is the mirror is helping me build a positive self- image, and that increases my confidence.

Another great trick I've learned: Magic Lipstick.

As any small town woman can tell you, if you go to town without your makeup on, you'll see everyone you know. Yet, some days there just isn't time. That's when I reach for the Magic Lipstick. One glance in the mirror tells me my no-makeup face looks shabby; then the lipstick goes on. All the difference in the world, I tell myself. I am then ready to confidently face the masses.

Projection is the tool that creates how others perceive you. Project yourself as confident and attractive and you will be amazed how many people accept your projection. Yet, beauty is in the eye of the beholder.

May you, like me, be blessed with an abundance of beautiful-eyed friends.

There is the other side of projection to consider, projecting yourself as self- conscious and uncomfortable with your appearance. Nothing will get you noticed faster. I suppose it's natural.

If you are uncomfortable about your appearance, we can't help wondering why. Not only are you projecting a negative image, but also self-consciousness encourages a closer, critical inspection, which most of us do not want.

I recently met a man who had a habit of tucking his chin. I assumed he had some neck difficulties but as we got acquainted, I learned long ago he had surgery on his jaw that did not go well and left him with a lot of scarring. Instinctively, he was tucking his chin to hide his scars. Doing so detracted from what a nice looking man he was, scars and all.

Yet scars do more than affect our appearance. They can stir bad memories. They can feel like a branded scarlet letter that we wish we could cover, yet, cannot. Or, like Quint in Jaws, scars can be badges of courage we wear with pride.

For most of us, our scars are a bit of all of these. To build confidence, we need to accept our scars. We need to stop seeing them as separate or something that happened to us, and begin seeing them as a part of us.

With this acceptance, we can find balance. We are then simply ourselves, not ourselves that something happened to, not our old self/new self, but just us. Accepting our scars makes us whole.

I'll admit that accepting scars is not easy. For some it may be a lifetime process. Yet that doesn't mean we should waver from the goal. Nor does it mean we can't fake it.

As I discussed previously, I generally wear a smile, whether in the mood or not. I tried the same with my appearance. I may not have felt confident. Yet, I put my shoulders back and marched into the room anyway and I was pleased with my reception.

A stumbling block for those with facial differences is photographs. While we can project confidence and beauty in the animated world, somehow, the split second of a photo can capture all the wrong stuff. To help, develop photo poses as you work with your face. That way, when a camera comes out, you quickly, instinctively, are in a pose that is your best.

Have several poses, so you don't always appear the same. Tipping your head can help soften an asymmetrical face. Do not refuse photographs. It isn't fair to your loved ones or to you. Step up to the camera and give it your best. When a friend shows you his great shot of you, smile and say thank you, even if you hate the photograph. Let the moment be captured. Later, you'll be glad you did. Besides, no one likes the party pooper who refuses to have photographs taken.

If a photo is particularly bad, ask to have your image removed, but make these occasions few. To those who want to shoot close-ups, say no. In photographs, as in life, be flexible, yet protective, of your appearance.

CHAPTER 21

Emerging From the Trenches

I had hoped this last chapter would be very upbeat and send you off with wings on your heals. Yet as I contemplated the subject, I doubted I could pull that off. Yes, emerging from the trenches is wonderful. No more planning the next procedure, or fretting the end result. Yet for me, leaving was difficult too.

I spent a lot of time there. I became friends with my comrades in arms. The trenches were familiar; maybe not home, but a place I survived. I was challenged, sometimes to my limits. In the trenches, I found strength I never knew I possessed. I was called a hero. Some of my proudest moments took place there, many of my worst nightmares, too. How do you walk away from such a place?

Of the volumes of journaling that I wrote during my healing odyssey, "Emerging from the Trenches" was perhaps my most common subject.

It was a huge transition, a lot to endure, a lot to think about. There were changes in me: wisdom, fear, new strengths and weaknesses. In the battlefield of my surgeries, I was assaulted, healed and planned the next attack—a harsh life. The everyday life of home was gentle, a welcoming place beyond those surgical battles.

Yet in the beginning, it was difficult to adjust to everyday life. After fighting so long, it was difficult to trust peace. Perhaps, too, a part of me missed the excitement of battle.

I think another reason I wrote so much about emerging from the trenches is because it is something you do alone. No matter how involved and helpful your loved ones are, emerging from the trenches is a solo task. Loved ones' compassion is a great help, but only you understand the days your memories won't stop pulling you back, or why another day you adamantly refuse to discuss anything that happened to you.

When contemplating this dilemma, I often thought back to the movie, "The Best Years of Our Lives," a story about soldiers returning from WWII. When away at war, the men longed for home but when they returned, they felt they didn't fit in—a limbo of transition. Time was needed to adjust. Though not as dire as war, the trenches of surgery aren't that different.

Give yourself time. Be patience.

Just like the soldiers of war, do not be surprised by haunting memories. As I stated in regard to my accident, twice within a few days' time I thought I would bleed to death. The first time was at the batting cage, the second was days later when packing was removed from my nose, and I lost over a pint of blood. For years, a deep emotional scar haunted me.

The damage to my nose and sinuses led to many severe nosebleeds, and in the beginning, a nosebleed would send me into a panic attack, my heart pounding with the terror of bleeding.

As time went on, I was able to soothe my emotional response, but it took years before a nosebleed didn't send my blood pressure through the roof.

There are other scars and memories that sneak back. Be ready to endure them. When I wrote the chapter "Making the Most of Your Appearance," I had forgotten about the shame and anguish I felt attending my son's graduation without a contact to cover my eye. Remembering was hurtful and I spent some time looking back and comforting myself.

When bad memories surface, do not turn away. If you run, you are adding the power of fear to them. If you ignore them, you are trivializing and dismissing the battles you fought. I remember the anger and frustration I felt when a woman said to me, "I just want this to be over for you."

It is never "over."

Though we move forward, our past is part of the building blocks of who we are today; pain and sadness are some of those blocks, but so are growth and healing. All of them wrapped together make our unique self.

While there is need to accept and deal with hurt from the past, there is also need to live life in the present, as unhindered as possible. Finding balance is part of the healing process.

When I felt I was becoming self-absorbed, I tried to "love thy neighbor" and turn my attention to helping others. If I felt caught in the rush of every day and missed life's depth, I turned to contemplation and prayer. When the "thinking about it too much" mode hit, it was time for a night out.

For me, especially in the beginning, emerging from the trenches and balancing the scars of the past with the present, was a tightrope walk, always needing adjustment. I preferred seeking that balance alone, but if you feel stuck, especially in depression, get help. Just make sure your helpers are moving you forward.

Accepting the past and fitting it into life is important, yet it is the past. We live in the present.

I have only been to one group therapy. It was for people with head injury and seizures. To me, it was a bitch session of self-centered people trying to outdo each other in "poor me." Not that each person didn't have very real difficulties and equally real anger and frustration to vent, yet, I found the session to be one of dear Aunt Rose's circle stories— an unending complaint without solution.

I often think back to the opening pilot of Star Trek's *Deep Space Nine*, in which Captain Sisko is a recent widower who keeps returning to the scene of his wife's death. He is asked repeatedly by aliens attempting to communicate with him: "Why do you exist here?"

At first, Captain Sisko is baffled, and cannot figure out why the aliens keep returning him to that horrible moment, but he eventually realizes that he is the one doing it. He is living in the past. Only he can make that tragic moment remain in the past, while he moves forward, living in the present.

How long will it take to emerge from the trenches—months, years? It is a matter unique to the individual. My best advice: don't rush it. Like healing, it isn't something to simply get past. Let it be a journey, difficult but powerful and enlightening.

Healing and emerging from the trenches can afford opportunities to learn. As you understand yourself, you can understand others, too. As you learn to be patient with yourself, your empathy for others can grow.

When you look in the mirror and, for the first time, don't feel a jolt of unfamiliarity, you can realize gratitude beyond what you expected. There is much knowledge to gain; why rush through?

Don't be surprised if sunsets now stun you with a beauty you never saw before. Allow yourself to live life with new depth. Change is the only constant. You are emerging from the trenches a changed person. Explore and embrace the new you.

I think this has turned out upbeat, after all. Not in a simple, chocolate cake sort of way, but in life's way, moving ever forward.

We have come so far. Let's celebrate!

THE END

Appendix

Selected Journals entries and correspondence

August 4, 1996

Today I am afraid.

I called Dr. Ridgway (primary care doctor) and he will take a look at me. I'm fine. I'm sure of it. It's just that as the swelling drains downward, my eye lid became more swollen than yesterday. My nose is bleeding a bit, too, probably also a result of drainage.

Everything is fine. I'm sure of it. Yet I am afraid.

August 5, 1996

The second worst day of my life.

I went to Grand Junction to have packing in my nose removed- and I was drowning in blood.

They managed to stop the bleeding, but crimany, what did they expect? This artery and my nose should have been taken care of last week when my eye surgery was done.

I am so angry!

And I never saw a doctor, only a physician's assistant and nurses aid who works in an ear/nose/throat clinic and didn't know what cephredene is. Where do these people get off? And the worst thing is, they are the only game in town.

Now I have this outrageous stuffed nose, pain and I missed an eye appointment.

I could scream! This packing is driving me crazy. It's way too much. I've pulled some out and I need to stop. No more gushers today, please!

Tomorrow I see "the doctor". It's going to be hard to be civil. But I don't want to Tee off the surgeon, do I? I need to be blunt, though. This all seems unprofessional to me. And I want to know what the radiologist said.

Is my nose as severely broken as I think? And if so, why this packing crap? I want answers. I do not trust this guy. I need to make this clear to him so that I can make educated guesses. Is there someone in Montrose? I need to find out.

I have some control. I need to find out how much, use it wisely, be Orthodox in my dealings and get the job done right!

AUGUST 27, 1996

As I looked at myself in the mirror, gazing at my odd shaped eye and scars along my nose, I began thinking these are not really scars, but a marking. It shows that on July 28, 1996, my Lord allowed me to continue my life on earth. It marks the day Ryan Todd was allowed to keep his mother beside him.

On that special day, it was noted Allen Todd would not be a widower. To brush so near death - shouldn't one be marked? I pray that each time I look in the mirror, I am reminded of this precious, wonderful gift of life.

September 2, 1996

Depression is getting hold of me. I have fought it valiantly all this time, but now I feel it pushing through. With it comes the worry of phobias too, but worst of all is the depression itself. I must not become defeated.

Five weeks have passed and still I am not seeing more than shadows from my left eye. Surgery is scheduled for Sept 11 but I do not want it.

I dread it

There is the possibility that I will need to spend 10 days in Denver - if my retina is torn. Most of that time I would be alone. I am terrified of how deeply depressed I might get.

Depression is such an ugly, bottomless pit. I cannot fall into it.

I fear I will never come back.

December 8, 1996

During my post accident surgeries, I told my friend Margaret that I was meeting my doctor in Grand Junction to pick (ie: choose) my nose. Nothing slips by that woman.

This song was born.

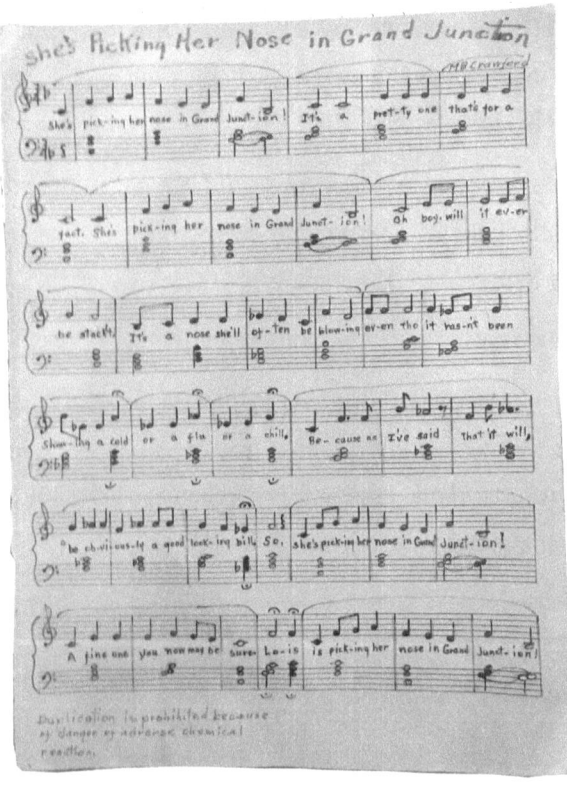

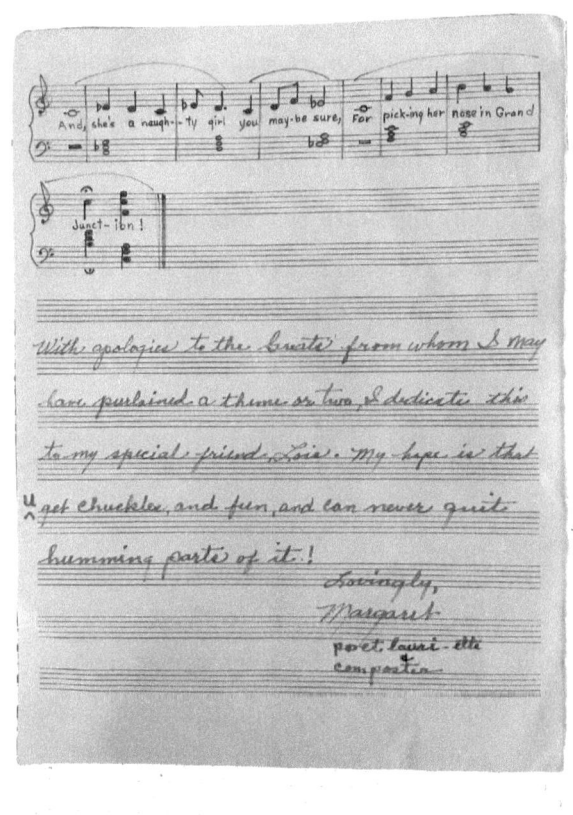

With apologies to the Greats from whom I may
have purloined a theme or two, I dedicate this
to my special friend, Lois. My hope is that
get chuckles, and fun, and can never quit
humming parts of it.!

Lovingly,
Margaret

poet, lauri-ette
compostia

February 5, 1997

If I had not been born with the name Hawk, it might have been easier. For as long as I remember, that name meant strength and independence, but mostly uniqueness. Hawks are unique. They fly alone.

That is why the sharp nose and equally sharp light eyes seemed to fit me so well. They were a Hawk's. I have a long line of curmudgeon cowboys and sharp tongued women to attest to this. People used to say I was pretty, but I think if was more likely I thought I was pretty and they did not want to argue with me. Those sharp, unique features winning the day again.

That is why, in a way, the deformity is easier to take than the reconstruction. At least the deformity; the sinking in of my eye, the deep scar on my nose, the large, odd angle of my pupil;. is unique. The reconstruction brings a simple, every day nose, like everyone else's and the colored contacts make my eyes a Barbie blue that only insecure women wear.

Where is the eye color of the sharp tongued Hawk women who drove off husband after husband and seemed no worse for wear? Where is the sharp, angular nose that led curmudgeons into fist fights well into their seventies?

Who are the women who go voluntarily to the knife so they can look like everyone else? Shouldn't we send them to therapy, instead of surgery?

If it is true that preservation of self is more important than self preservation, shouldn't plastic surgeons find a way to return us to our original selves instead of fluffed up Barbie dolls that imitate us?

The Hawk becomes a common sparrow, a creature perhaps more beautiful with its soft angles and whimsical aerobatics, but common, none the less.

January 7, 1997

I have seen my ugliness.

One of the photos we took for our Christmas card showed it plainly - an eye misshapen, distorted, reminding me of Quasimodo. On a face somewhat pretty, it is startling. I see my ugliness in others faces. Since my hair was beaded, I now get the true stares - a disfigurement, an oddity, horrible yet unable to look away from.

I see my ugliness in the mirror. I look full at my face, not just the damaged eye, and I see the asymmetry, also the way I used to look; my unmatched eyes now mocking a beauty that once was. I see the damage, the disfigurement, the pain and my heart weeps for anyone who must carry such a loathsome burden. Then I look again and it is me.

Why am I out? Why am I not veiled? How do I, why do I, let others endure the sight of me? I am ugly, revolting.

I smile a confident smile and much of the disfigurement disappears, yet it is always there, cloaked by a fragile, tentative shell that may at any time collapse and leave an ugly, morbid woman in disgrace.

God help me.

February 6, 1997

It is like waking up one morning and finding all your clothes have been replaced by others that aren't you and look, in part, hideous, yet you have no choice. This is now your wardrobe. Every piece of clothing has a tear or rip, either near the breast or the hip, and though it is embarrassing, you must wear them. You never know who will notice. Most people glance at the tears and take them in as remnants of a bad day. Yet others stare, mortified, embarrassed whether for you, for themselves or both, you do not know.

March 25, 1998

Thoughts on an Injured Life

Scandalized and vandalized
All true and well written
Numerized and scrutinized
Where did the bright girl go?
Summarized and theorized
She must be here some place
Galvanized and de-energized
Can she make it through court?
Face pounded
Heavy chisel
Mind bent
IQ fizzle
Keep smiling
Doctor waiting
My day in court.

OCTOBER 14, 2008

My year in a holding pattern is up. Time again to seek a scalpel. I've found a new plastic surgeon, Dr. Menick, a true mucky muck. Of all the plastic surgeons in the US, my dermatologist recommended two – he is one of them.

The trick now is to convince him I am worthy of his services. I sent him an E mail; raw information about my face, but a few well chosen bits of humor, too. I want to catch his attention, intrigue him. Today I had a facial so I would look my best for the camera. Of course, my best is also my worst - highlight my imperfections to heighten his interest, let him ponder the possibilities of change. One picture was of me truly trying to look my best; make-up on, big smile, head tipped slightly to the left to mask the asymmetry of my eyes. I'm pulling out all the tricks – entice to slice.

December 28, 2008

Knight Boogie

He is my knight in shining armor.

He will pull the wicked witch's mask from me.

He will lift me from my bed of long, fitful slumber and I will arise whole and free.

He is my boogie man.

He will rip into me, twist me, slice me, bruise me and try as I might I cannot flee from him.

He is my surgeon and it is time to meet his knife.

February 4, 2009

Thought you'd like a surgery update: That Dr. Me-nick is a genius. While I'm not yet seeing most of the changes in my face (still pretty swollen) I'm feeling them. My forehead is far looser and no longer has that glued down feel on the scar tissue.   My eye brow is now where the eye brow should be, relieving a lot of tension as well. The nerve bundle (like shingles) that has been on my brow since flap down surgery (2 ½ years ago) has greatly dissipated and hopefully will go away (yes!)

The tip of my nose feels like the tip of my nose. Prior, it was like having a sock on that's twisted. It pulls and tugs at your leg but when you straighten it, everything feels smooth. (Yeah, like that.) The large scar on the side of my nose is gone and thus no longer protrudes into my nasal passage. (Don't want to go into detail on the inner workings of my nasal passage, but let's just say nose picking is smooth sailing these days! – OOOO – sorry couldn't resist – the comment, not the nose picking- no, that's not what I meant; I can resist nose picking – oh, never mind.)

Dr. Menick took ear cartilage to build my nostril and it's weird how much better it feels. Before, my nostril was like a tent made out of light cotton. Now I've got a sturdy canvas nostril and it feels solid. The one difference I already see is from the incision going down the side of my cheek which took out excess skin. At first I couldn't figure out why Dr. Menick went so far down my face, nearly to the chin. Then I saw it. He made a smile line to match the right side. He thinks of everything!

A frigging genius!

OCTOBER 3, 2011

Emerging from the Trenches

I am at the stage, or nearly there, when I emerge from the trenches.

I am battle worn, thread bare, hero, coward – all this and so much more. I think of the movie The Best Years of Our Lives. Yes, that is me. I, too, am a soldier, but the bombs that explode around me are disfigurement. My gun fire comes from a surgeon's knife.

In the trenches, I adjust to this harsh life quickly. After all it is my third tour of duty. The first thing I learned was to live each moment fully because I didn't know what the next moment might bring. When I laughed, I knew to laugh hard. My tears were rich. Some of the most brilliant moments of my life were there in the trenches.

But mostly it was dark and frightening. Hard to keep up morale. No slacking or I would surely die.

There is great pride when emerging from the trenches.

I have survived bloody battles, war whoops and hanging my head in the rain. I begged God to make it all stop because I couldn't go on and then I did go on. I emerge alive. Exhilarated.

Yet leaving the trenches is not easy. Upon its completion, this last tour of duty will have lasted more than three years. Three years of battle plans, charges and retreats.

How do you walk away from that?

And there is the fear that it will not walk away from me. Just months before my cancer diagnosis, I was telling a new optometrist about my accident. Suddenly my heart raced and I wanted to scream "leave me alone".

I recognized the reaction almost immediately – post traumatic stress disorder. And if an accident whose recovery took one year and with better results ended in PTSS, what could two tours of duty with lesser results bring? And then the soldier in me steps forward.

She reminds me that at this moment there is no battle. She says that fight may never come, and if it does, we will battle it then – and be victorious. She is a good soldier.

Leaving the trenches means returning to civilian life, but this soldier's life of wounds and fears, does not compute well in the everyday. "I want this to be over for you," one friend repeated so many times I had to insist she stop.

Over?

This is never over. I may emerge from the trench but the battle scars come with me. And while I relish the idea of life outside the trenches, do I want to push those years away like some disruption that should be forgotten?

As ugly and difficult as my accident and this cancer odyssey have been, it is a powerful part of my life. It is an important part of who I am. And then an unexpected ambush from friendly fire; my current battles called unnecessary and frivolous.

The wound sears deep. I stagger. The soldier in me arises again.

"Head up and eye on your goal", she says. "You're almost out of the trenches. Don't you let anything get in your way."

"Aye, sir," I say.

I am a good soldier.

NOTES

Notes

Notes

NOTES

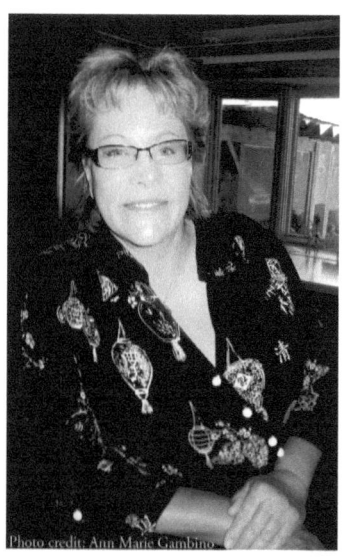

Photo credit: Ann Marie Gambino

Lois Hawk Todd was born and raised in Lebanon, Oregon where she grew up with a deep love and appreciation of the great outdoors.

In 1976, at age nineteen, she packed her worldly possessions into her car and drove off to explore America. Her travels took her to western Colorado, where she has resided ever since.

In 1981, she graduated from Mesa College in Grand Junction, Colorado with an associates degree in early childhood education. She married her husband, Allen Todd, in 1983 and in 1986 her son, Ryan Todd, was born.

In 1996, Lois was struck by a baseball that shattered her face. Her experiences after the accident led her to write this book.

Lois has always enjoyed writing. She has been employed as a journalist and has published poetry. Via her company, Perplex Murder Mystery Games, she wrote and saw performed thirty-four interactive murder mystery games.

An avid traveler, Lois keeps a bag half-packed at all times. Her travels have taken her near and far. To date, she has visited fifteen countries outside the United States.

Lois also enjoys cooking and gardening. She is an enthusiastic fan of Star Trek and is known to her Trekkie friends as "Lt. Lois."

Lois resides with her husband in Paonia, Colorado.